Shedding that which is Not Us
A Working-Class Guide to Life Foods
Training and Healing
By Danny Shaw

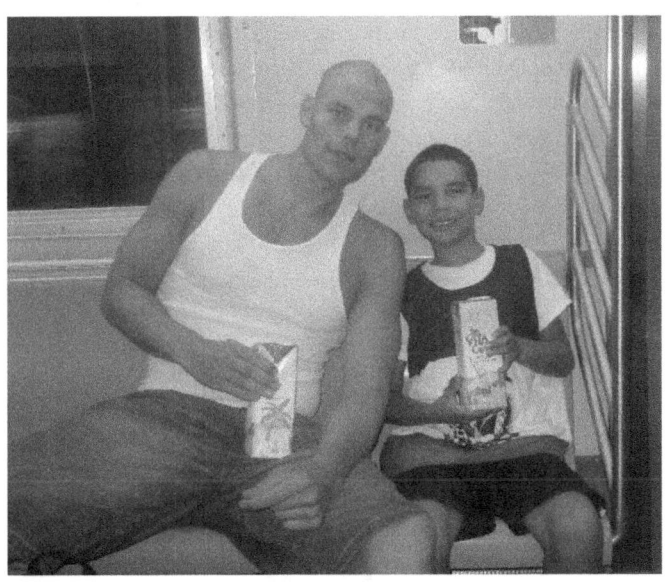

Internationalist Training Publications
For information regarding this book contact Danny Shaw
Columbia on Facebook or at DRS33@Columbia.edu

By Danny Shaw

Shedding that which is not Us
365 Days of Resistance: Standing on the Shoulders
of Giants
The Saints of Santo Domingo: Dominican
Resistance in the Age of Neocolonialism
Paisajes de Amor y Combate
Diving over Infinite Horizons
My Son Blazes within Me: So Many Contradictions,
So Little Time

Dedicated to Ernesto Rafael:
Your curiosity and smile
radiate out warmth, love and sensitivity
to a world in dire need of it.
Keep building up your wide-eyed inquisitive mind
and an impenetrable self-love and love of life.
(And try to eat healthy. I know it's tough.)
I will always be proud of you, young lad and will be
here for you no what tribulations you confront.
The world is yours to reinvent!

Dedicated to my mother:
for transforming unspeakable pain into love
and putting the writing of George Jackson, Assata
Shakur, Bobby Sands, John Brown and so many
others into my hands.

Dedicated to my sister Jennifer:
For all of the kindness and affection
you have shared with a world
which rarely reciprocated your warmth.

Dedicated to Doc Precise:
Patrice, the People's Chemist
aka "The Booch Killa"
The synthesis of Discipline and loyalty
Jamaica, Queens and Trinidad
Love and the streets.

Table of Contents

x

Introduction

As a student, practitioner and chef of Life Foods living, I strive to grow younger every day. At thirty-eight, I feel lighter and younger than I did at twenty-one or twenty-eight or at any age for that matter. I want to share my story with you and the steps I took to emerge as the Life Foods chef, boxer, yogi, professor, father, runner, author, mentor and revolutionary that I am today. What follows is a combination of storytelling, testimony, autobiography, nutritional analysis and what motivated this book in the first place — my own recipes that I used to destarchify. Here within, I share what I put into my tank to achieve supreme training results, a high amount of energy and production and maximum whole brain functioning.

What does Life Foods consist of?

The premise of Life Foods — a school of nutrition founded by Dr. David Jubb and Annie Padden Jubb — is that the best foods for our minds, our bodies and our environment are fruits, vegetables, seeds, sprouts and nuts. These are living foods in nature and have their life force and digestive enzymes intact. Eating these Life Foods facilitates the digestive process, freeing up energy for the brain and central nervous system to function at optimum capacity. We do not use dairy, meat, or any cooked food. Cooking food kills the digestive enzymes and alters the chemical structure of the food. What animal in history has ever used a stove besides us humans? My journey has taught me that as I let go of cooked food I was able to experience life more vividly. What could radically altering your sustenance do for you?

Unlike veganism, Life Foods living discourages the consumption of rice, oats or any grains. Life Foods also limits the consumption of legumes such as chickpeas, beans or lentils. Both grains and legumes are strange indigestible proteins that are taxing on the liver and gall bladder and can cause degenerative effects on brain and digestive functioning over time. As many people can testify, beans can cause flatulence and distention.

Life Foods differs from Raw Foods because it rejects "starchy hybrid foods with runaway sugars such as potatoes, rice, corn, wheat, all grain-flour products, all tuberous vegetables like carrots, beets, commercial bananas and dates. Other hybrids to avoid, especially by those healing cancer, are commercially grown strawberries, pineapples, mushrooms, kiwi and soybeans."[1] Organic versions

---

[1] Annie Padden Jubb and Dr. David Jubb's <u>Lifefood Recipes Book Living on Life Force</u> provides a more complete explanation of this nutritional school of thought which grows

of these fruits are still fine. Hybrids are foods that are man-made, meaning that have been cross bred over time. According to Dr. Jubb's microscopic investigation, these selectively bred items are not as easily absorbed as cellular fuel and are spit back out into the bloodstream in the form of indigestible runaway sugars.

A basic premise is that less is more for the body. By saying no to harmful foods, through proper Life Foods fasting, the body can heal itself from any manifestation of dis-ease. Say goodbye to indigestion, heartburn, stomachaches, headaches, acid reflux, gastritis, ulcers, constipation, gout, diarrhea, nausea, and fatigue. The key to health is digestion. All these unnatural conditions are localized expressions of the reality that we are introducing harmful things to our bodies and overburdening our digestive track.

At first glance, I can relate to how unrealistic and austere this must appear to the average American. When I first learned about natural healing, I dismissed it as some crazy, bizarre hippie thing. I want to share with you my story and what elevated me to where I am today. I would not approach Life Foods as if you are going straight to step 10. It took me years of experimenting and zigzagging to get to

out of Ann Wigmore's Living Foods movement. Berkeley: North Atlantic Books. 2003.

where I am today. In another ten years, I hope to graze previously undiscovered lands. We never stop growing. Life is not a linear path but rather a dialectical maze where we learn from our missteps and continue to push forward. Take your first steps at your own pace. Even if you only take away a few life-lessons from this book, you will be taking steps in the right direction. You cannot go wrong. You have nothing to lose but your gastric chains!

Section I. My Journey: The Starch Withdrawal

I never thought I would be capable of adopting a plant- and fruit-based lifestyle. I was an absolute *starchoholic*. I grew up a big kid, loving all types of "classic American" meals. Thursday was pasta and meatball night with the basketball team. On Saturdays, we visited my aunt and uncle for hamburgers and beans. On Sunday mornings, my uncle prepared a family classic called "Eggs in the Hole," which consisted of fried bread, draped in fried eggs, cheese and bacon. Sunday afternoons brought elaborate roast pork and roast beef family dinners at my nana's house. Since I didn't like roast pork, my family lied to me and told me it was chicken and gave me a bottle of ketchup so that I didn't complain.

My mother was a waitress and bartender. She brought home leftovers such as meat pizzas and steak and cheese subs from the bar. When my mom was away at work, I heated up fish sticks and burgers.

To this day, my mouth waters with nostalgia just remembering these moments. For the son of a single mother, "good food" signified good cheer, a close knit-family and stability. Some of my best childhood memories are of the family going out to Chilis, "Chinese" food restaurants, BBQ spots, and IHOP, the International House of Pancakes. As early as six- or seven-years-old, I developed a habit my family members still tease me about. Not only did I lick my plate clean, but I also licked others' plates clean, often before the unsuspecting victims had finished their meal.[2] As my older siblings told me years later, it turns out my father had a penchant for finishing off others' meals as well.

But does family and social time have to be synonymous with stuff your face time? Would I have made it past forty-five at this rate? How many medications are my family members on today?

My maternal grandfather died at fifty-nine from his third heart attack. My uncle had a quadruple bypass at thirty-nine and another at fifty-nine. My cousins have diabetes and hypoglycemia. My aunts and mother suffer from a seemingly endless assortment of maladies. My father died of lung cancer at sixty-one.

As a typical kid and teenager, I indulged in overeating like most young people in this country. For the first twenty-five years of my life, I had no sense that there was even an option to digestive discomfort. I thought of vegans as strange, scrawny, odd-ball white people who lived far away from where I did.

---

[2] Belated apologies to Ben, Josh, Ernesto, Karina and all my other traumatized acquaintances who suffered in the path of my wanton starchaholicism.

I paid the price for eating the Standard American Diet (SAD). I developed problems with hypoglycemia. My mother rushed to give me a candy bar in an attempt to "balance my blood sugar" at basketball games. I endured extreme constipation. I remember family conventions aimed at figuring out how to get me to go the bathroom. After eating, I felt horrible tummy aches and chest pain. In high school, I got skin peals on my face because my acne was so bad. I was on track to endure a great deal of suffering. And this is coming from a young man who was the captain of one of the best High School basketball teams in New England, Brockton High. I can relate to what other young people are suffering through — often times in silence — and it breaks my heart.

One afternoon, just recently, after football practice, my thirteen-year-old son made himself a triple decker burger bathed in cheese and bacon. I remember those days of being young and carefree. People often ask me if my son, Ernesto Rafael follows my lifestyle. I don't believe I can force Ernesto into a rhythm that he does not voluntarily embrace. He has entered into his stage of rebellion against the established order, which in our home is Life Foods. I do regular check-ins with my Ernesto to see how he is feeling but I want him to find his own way and arrive at his own conclusions. At the same time, I feel a great deal of ambivalence and sadness because I know he is addicted to the poisons 99% of our children have become addicted to.

According to conventional wisdom aka the "doctors" and the "experts," Ernesto and I are doomed to experience the same anguish as our family members because "dis-ease runs in the genes." Inspired not to repeat the mistakes of my kin, I opened my mind up to alternative ways of living.

I was fortunate my mother taught me how to think critically and to question every source of information. My nutritional pilgrimage served as an analogy for my intellectual, spiritual and ideological search in this society. The answers were not readily available, nor were they easy realities to accept. I had to dig. I had to dare to rebel because it is right to rebel!

The Vegan Gut: Transcending Veganism

In my mid 20's, I started shifting towards eating "leaner meats" and integrating more greens into my diet. A conscious girlfriend — who was a dancer, rapper, poet, life rebel and yogi — introduced me to a more peaceful way of co-existing with the world. I pinpoint those Johnny Cash stretching sessions and conversations with her about healing as the first time I thought about nutrition. My mother tried to instill some of this in me but let's face it: We are never prophets in our own land. My mother's wisdom fell on deaf ears. As I discussed, my Ernesto has a similar response to my lifestyle today.

With time and a lot of experimentation, I moved towards vegetarianism and eventually veganism. But I saw that even though I was a boxer and was working out a great deal, I was still a very big, big guy. I was 6' 6 and weighed 245 lbs. Even if I was boxing four or five times a week and running twenty to thirty miles, I still had a belly. I searched within: "How can I have a gut if I am eating almost all vegan?" I was erroneously equating veganism with healing. I came to the conclusion that all of the starches I was consuming — like plantain, bread, rice and soy — were not allowing me to shed that which was not me.

I had the vegan belly![3]
I was a Big Boy Vegan.

I have a lot of love for my vegan family but justifying eating potato-chips and french-fries because no animals are hurt in the process did not make sense to me. This lifestyle is an ethical

---

[3] Throughout the book, I return to slogans that I coined as I interacted with an increasing amount of people who wanted to heal. I centered and italicized these concepts because they are the pillars of what I believe and read as a roadmap of my spiritual world outlook.

approach to all of the life that abounds in nature but what about your life? I sought to discover what was the most nutritionally-sound way to live?

Transcending veganism was a big step for me. But it was not easy and it took a lot of support. In the spring of 2009, I came into contact with some of the most eccentric, disciplined, off-the-grid nutritionists you could ever imagine. As I would learn for myself, studying and adopting their Life Foods lifestyle would change who I was forever.

Forever Humbled, Forever Grateful

I was introduced to Thomas the Cleanser who is known in the Life Foods world as Raining Horse. He offered to be my *Phoenix Fastician*.[4] "What the *!#$%* is that?" I wondered. Initially, I thought the Cleanser was "out there." He smelled like castor oil, the earth and he had a trampoline in his kitchen. I bumped into him several more times at neighborhood workout sessions in Harlem hosted by an organization called *Revolutionary Fitness*.

The Cleanser was lean, active and had a certain harmonious glow about him. My curiosity was heightened. What was the secret to his high energy?

---

[4] Dr. Jubb calls the healers he has trained Phoenix Fasticians.

The Cleanser hosted dinners on 135th St. after the work outs where he served papaya based smoothies, steamed veggies and homemade nut milks. In the beginning, it was all rather strange. Some of it was actually grotesque. One night, he served a group of us a so called "dessert." It was sea minerals on top of orange slices. I looked over at three of my fellow travelers, Ben, Karina and Juan Pablo. They were equally horrified. I thought we were all going to get sick. The minerals were a mix of sea vegetables blended into a fine green powder. Just as peanut butter can stick to the top of your mouth, the sea weed and ocean smell stuck to the roofs of our mouths and overwhelmed us. We jostled to be the first one into the bathroom to spit it out. We endured what we perceived as a most frightening experience! The Cleanser just peered over us with his wry grin and asked, "Isn't that delicious?" There was a disconnect between where the mentor and the mentees where at.

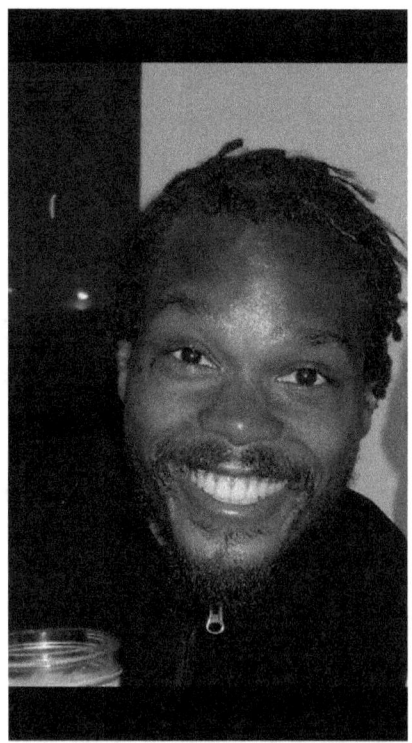

Thomas the Cleanser, the Urban Dove with the Life Foods glow

To this day, our coterie of friends laughs at these original dinners and the Cleanser's cutting-edge style. He was ahead of his time. But ultimately, this was exploration and discovery; I felt light and sharp after the Cleanser's meals. Everything flowed through me smoothly. I observed that Thomas was living life in another dimension and on another level of intensity. I was determined to learn more.

The Cleanser and I grew closer. He was a gastro-intestinal genius, citing theories about healing and teaching me about the intricacies of the human body. I took it all in, jotting down notes on his elaborate studies. With an encyclopedic recall of knowledge and an unmatched glowing positivity, he now had my attention. He asked me "Do you want to take it to the next level?" I thought *why not challenge myself and do a weekend cleanse?*

On a Thursday night, he walked seven miles in his five toe vibrams from 89th St. in Manhattan to the South Bronx with a bag of Brazil nuts, a case of Kombucha, coconut oil, and organic lemons, apples and pears. He didn't believe in subways or any form of modern transportation. I am not sure whether it was because of his Ludite convictions or the fact that he did not have a dollar to his name, but he walked the three hours — with pounds of produce under his arm — to get to my apartment. He told me he would be there by 8 p.m. He arrived at 1 a.m. He proudly smelled of castor oil which he had put all over his body to promote internal healing. As I learned, Life Foodists are never on time. They say: "Time does not exist; All that exists is now." Because I had to be up to teach at John Jay College by 7 a.m. I explained that time did indeed exist, for me at least, and that we could start the next morning.

With his supplies of Castor Oil Pacts and Life Water (see Section IV), the Cleanser set up shop in my apartment. He swept the cupboards clean of pasta, honey bunches of oats, wheat bread, soy products and the other canned and boxed starches. He stayed with me like a friend does for someone detoxing off Percocets or Heroin. He showed me an incredible patience and affection as he walked me through my withdrawal from starches.

Destarchifying

There are two types of carbohydrates, those that grow in nature and those that are man-made and are loaded with chemical additives. These are called complex and refined carbohydrates, respectively. Whole wheat and white rice are some of the most common complex carbs that unsuspectingly contribute to nagging health problems. An autopsy may indicate that a death was caused by a stroke or heart failure, but it would be more accurate if it read, "Death by starchicide and lifestyle."

One of the differentiating aspects of Life Foods from vegetarianism is expurgating processed starches from our lifestyle. These mucous-forming foods are a silent killer. This is where the unclogging and unseating of intestinal debris begins. This triggers a Healing Crisis!

A healing crisis is the releasing of the toxicity locked within. It is essential to have support during this reawakening period, so that you do not turn back and you can correctly interpret what is happening to your body. The healing crisis can manifest itself through headaches, an outpouring of mucus, cathartic trips to the bathroom, break-outs on the skin and other manifold manifestations of internal cleansing. Though this sounds alarming, this is the withdrawal, the rehabilitation and the forging of your freedom. The body is clearing away mold, fungus and yeast.

The healing crisis is in fact a healing nirvana.

These are the spiritually and physically empowering moments that will mark your journey. Embrace them, don't run from them. While initially these will be rough-and-tumble moments, you will soon awake afresh, as if someone had come in the middle of the night and granted you a new body.

Goose bumps surface every time I think about The Cleanser and I building in my kitchen, trekking through this labyrinth called life. As schmaltzy as it sounds, it was like I was the chosen one. There was pressure on the Cleanser, from the top of the Life Foods hierarchy, to charge me $350 dollars for the weekend of guided cleansing. But the Cleanser allowed me to give what I was able to. I was open and he shared with me. To this day he embodies the spirit of what we seek to do with Life Foods — help others heal so that they can take control back over their health. This mentality stands in stark contrast to the spiritual materialism that has taken root across this country with self-proclaimed gurus trying to make a buck off people's pain. We have to meet people where they are at. Otherwise, we are effectively abandoning them amidst a war that we are losing.

I could not have done it without The Cleanser's support, camaraderie and expertise. I felt the toxins exiting my body. I was like an overworked, over-stretched laborer who suddenly hit the lottery and was finally free from toil to pursue a long-lost dream.

I haven't looked back since. After 26 days, I felt the last traces of starches and mucus leave my body.

My first Healing Crisis was complete!

This was my introduction to Life Foods and what a journey it has been. Once I had learned to heal myself, I set out to help others heal, first in my immediate milieu, then far beyond. Today I am positioned to do for others, what The Cleanser did for me. This is both an honor and a responsibility. No one should have to suffer from being backed up and having nightmarish episodes of a leaky gut. We all have a doctor within!

Digestion 101: Evacuations

Dr. Jubb called bowel movements *Evacuations*. The first time I heard this euphemism, I thought it was hilarious. I always pause during workshops before I open up the topic of bowel movements. I ask the group if they are ready to broach this socially awkward or taboo topic which brings up both discomfort and lots of laughs.

Evacuations are a central measure of what we are trying to achieve. One of my nicknames, "The Evacuator" makes light of the fact that we are really going to get things moving. As you evacuate the old refuse that is holding you back, you will usher in a fresh, poignant, new you.

We want our nutrition to pass through us in a matter of hours, not days and certainly not weeks. How many minutes exactly is tough to say but studies indicate that when we juice it takes a matter of mere minutes to distribute the mineralization into the bloodstream. The odor and color of your poop reflects how long this gunk has been rotting away in your body. We want that out. In the words of Shrek: "Better out than in I always say."

Our lives depend on getting this built up waste out. The quicker we can remove the gunk, the better. You want your evacuations to be light and break away. There will not be any more long, hard captain's logs or egregious farting that sends your close family members running and ducking for cover. Darker colors and overwhelmingly pungent stenches are a sign that the food has begun to rot away within you. That is not to say that the poop of the cleansed smells of lavender essential oil, but it certainly does not have a malodorous scent of death which is a sure sign of constipation, a truly American epidemic. What a horrific feeling millions of Americas have to endure. There is nothing natural about this condition. This is completely unnecessary and reversible.

When you improve the treatment of your body, you will evacuate in the range of four times a day.[5] It may seem silly to treat this as scripture but a true healer's initial inquiry must address these very questions.

After completing a 21-day cleanse and a round of colonics, a MMA (Mixed Martial Arts) fighter told me: "Wow it feels so great to be *cleansed*." If only the process of unpacking decades of self-intoxication was so quick. When are we truly cleaned out or cleansed?

---

[5] There could be days where this shifts some of course. Life Water is going to promote super evacuations which are like liquefied nuclear bombs. I have gone up to 10 times with Life Water. But this must be used sparingly less we dehydrate ourselves. Only do this on a rest-active cycle.

There is no definitive answer for reaching Life Foods nirvana, as everybody, mind and spirit is unique. The science says that a 110-day Life Foods fast can starve out and remove the parasites. Dr. Jubb told me that a series of seven to ten Gall Bladder and Liver Flushes really digs up and does away with decades of compact fecal matter.

Considering we are surrounded by toxicity everywhere we turn, we should gently make the effort to live as healthy and pure as we can, taking into consideration each of our own unique challenges. Only if we were teleported out of The Toxic States of America back into nature — where fruits grow bountifully without the interference of man and chemicals and streams flow without being bottled up by Poland Spring — could we ever know what it means to live a pure life and be cleansed.

As I will discuss later, there are relatively untouched, natural havens in the world, from the Amazon to the lush jungles of the Philippines, where centenarians still dance to the tune of ancient rhythms and wisdom. It is this harmony with nature — what the Quechua people of the Andes call *sumac kawsay* — that we should seek to emulate.

We Need to Live-it, not Die-t.

We should seek to move beyond the concept of a "*die*-t". What a narrow, evil four-letter word! Dieting denotes self-deprivation and a temporary stage or fad to get a specific outcome. We have all heard friends say "Lawrence's wedding is coming up and I have to fit into this dress." But then what? What is outlined here is a new way to approach life in general. We need to *Live-it*, not Die-t. *Shedding that which is not Us* outlines the first steps towards living a purer life that this society has never taught us how to live.

The Pitfalls of Health Sectarianism

There are many "competing" theories in the nutritional world. Why should you follow this life style or another other particular nutritional worldview?

You should not adopt any information uncritically or blindly follow any program. You should explore, experiment and see what works for you. I am not a Health Sectarian. There are no competing schools of nutrition, there is only growth. It is good to scrutinize and try other healing programs and test new theories and ideas. I recently discovered the benefits of colonics in tandem with nutritional cleansing. Liquefied cleansing lifts debris up in the colon; colonics floods it out for good.

As long as you are following a program that works for you and the earth, you are on the right path. This is merely a roadmap to share some of my explorations.

With that said, there are nutritional programs out there that are misleading. It is worth surveying some of the other theories for healing up the gut that are popular today.

Dr. Peter J. D'Adamo's research suggests that one's blood type indicates what diet to follow. In *4 Blood Types, 4 Diets Eat Right for Your Type*, D'Adamo designs diets drawing from the following categories meats and poultry, oils and fats, nuts and seeds, cereals, breads and muffins, spices, herbal teas, vegetables, sea food, eggs and dairy.[6] He puts fourth that the idea that as long as you choose the right particular fish or spice you will be fine. He goes as far as condoning the use of white sugar for certain blood types. Feeding people what they want to hear, Dr. D'Adamo's "die-t" doesn't force you to give up any of the harmful food groups and their concomitant consequences. D'Adamo uses statistics and studies to feed people rubbish. I wish his findings were accurate. I mean who wouldn't want

---

[6] New York: G.P. Putnam's Sons. 1996.

a scientific justification for eating steaks, starches and candies? His argument does not require any sacrifice on the part of the participant.

In contrast, Life Foods is hard work. Life Foods is a gentle, allowing approach to a new lifestyle. If you already have it all figured out, if you are already convinced that the Standard American Diet (SAD) works for you, then you will be reading this book for pure entertainment purposes so that you can poke fun at us "madmen and mad women." We should all have a deep distrust of the dominant modalities of die-ting in the U.S. If you feel you are suffering more than you should and want to live pain free and inflammation free, Life Foods offers some amazing information and answers, in hopes that you can integrate this into your lifestyle.

The Atkins diet, the Paleo diet and the Omni diet posit that people should let go of all the processed starches but should continue to bring in some meat. In The Omni Diet, Registered Nurse Tana Amen outlines a 70% plant and 30% meat approach to healing.[7] These are great steps, perhaps for achieving your own personal training results, but this program will not usher in the healing and complete reboot that we need. Where do you want to be? Can you push it further? Maybe the Paleo or Omni balance is a temporary stage for you as you

---

[7] New York: St. Martin's Griffin. 2013.

begin to let go of that which was doing harm to you. It is important to take realistic steps for yourself. Even though hummus was not part of Life Foods it got me through tough moments; for others it was coffee or pea soup.

It is important to state that we are not super-humans. Sometimes a close friend will inspect my plate at a conference or public event to see if I have committed any infraction against the Life Foods gospel. This is overkill. Let me breathe and be. I am tempted everyday by fast food, school food, my sons' meals and all of the poison that surrounds us. I do my best to resist because I know what is right and best for my body. But every once in a while, I am too human and I break down, caving in to a scrumptious Indian, Italian or Thai meal.

It is very cute when someone just starting out inquires "Ooh and when can I cheat? What are my cheat days?" Cheating implies that there is something to diverge from. Establish that routine and then in dialogue with your body and the universe you will know when it is time to be allowing and to deviate a bit. But earn that right. Feel good about it.

We should not split hairs over relatively insignificant questions. Often, our detractors harp in on the most trivial detail, for example, our rejection of bananas because they have become genetically modified. Losing sight of the big picture, they seize the most outlandish belief or statement in order to discredit our entire world view.

We must not be too rigid unless that is what really works for you. What counts is not what you do in public moments to impress people. It is what you do in the private moments which account for 95% of your time.

If a bit of carrot juice, baked potato, hummus or a piece of fish here or there is your greatest nutritional transgression, you are on your way to living a long healthy life.

We have to be allowing. Don't jump into something that is so overwhelming that you are then going to hurl yourself back to past habits out of frustration. Be patient with yourself. What today appears impossible could one day become your lifestyle. Just keep pushing! In the words of the Vietnamese sage and independence leader, Ho Chi Minh: "Those who walk the road know it is hard. Scale one mountain and another appears. But once you mount the highest peak, 10,000 miles appear before your eyes."

The Dis-ease Establishment

Realize that there is a war being unleashed against our health every day in this country. Your starting point is that you are going to battle.

A simple drive down Route 95 or any highway or a leisurely stroll down any main street in any city in this country reveals the countless death foods which box us in. There are elite interests who want to strip us of control over our surroundings. They fear a self-determining people. A dependent *sheepelized* people will continue to consume their own doom. A healthy body is not a profitable body for the pharmaceutical industry. Defy them. Take control back.

I took a picture of my family's medicine cabinet. My nieces and nephews consume four, five or even more medications a day. When I gathered all of the "meds" together, the kitchen table was so crowded, there was no room left for anything else. This was symbolic of our plight as a besieged people. Never before in human history have a people faced such a drastic medical holocaust as that which is occurring before our eyes. It is scary to think that the generation my son belongs to may not outlive my generation. All of the carcinogenic chemicals introduced into our food signify an earlier death sentence for the generation coming of age today.

Monsanto's herbicide, Roundup, found in many conventional fruits and vegetables, has been found to cause cancer.[8]

Mark Schatzker's research in *The Dorito Effect: The Surprising New Truth about Food and Flavor* finds that "The birth of doritos was a watershed moment. Flavor wasn't up to Mother Nature anymore. Now it was in the hands of the folks in marketing."[9] For Schatzker, the dorito represents the replacement of real food with genetically altered food. Chemically induced flavoring is the wave of the future, a future sure to be dominated by earlier deaths from more cancer, diabetes, and drugs. The choice is not between healthy eating and traditional eating; it is between conscious eating and an agonizing death.

Apologists for the chemical holocaust argue that people are living longer today but what is the quality of their lives? They are dependent on chemicals. They chase around doctors to make infinite appointments to see this or that "specialist." Too busy surviving and chasing around the next pill to fill their voids, they have no time to live.

---

[8] Peeples, Lynn. "A Menacing Mix In Antibiotic Resistance: Herbicides, Heavy Metals And Factory Farms." *Huffington Post.* 3/24/2015

[9] New York: Simon and Schuster. 2015.

How can those responsible for the sickness then pretend to offer the cure? The very powerful interests who bombard us with advertisements for Applebee's buffalo wings, ranch dressing and beer, then broadcast commercials for Viagra and ACE inhibitors. As I will examine later in a section on cancer and the medical industry, many "specialists" are pompous charlatans who merely regurgitated their mis-training to get A+'s and promotions.

What a pack of lies! What a pack of pigs!

In the early 20th century, the Rockefellers, Mellons, Duponts and other ruling families ensured that there was zero nutritional, holistic training for doctors. Any school that did not abide by their parameters was denied licensing.[10] This was how they established a monopoly over "acceptable" and "unacceptable" medicine. Those genuine healers who refused to play the game were marginalized and labeled "quacks." This was the foundation of the monopoly over medicine that we witness today. The Disease Establishment fears, rejects and represses alternative medicine. The dominant medical paradigm offers no option to surgeries, pills, chemotherapy and radiation. Ultimately, it is up to us to organize for the overthrow of a failed

---

[10] For further treatment of this issue, see *The Truth about Cancer Part I.*

social system but in the meantime, we must collectively trill a different path forward!

Beyond liberation at the individual gut level, there is a more pressing liberation that we must address that involves a truly protracted struggle. I will address how collective and individual liberation are intertwined in the conclusion of this book, but suffice to say for now — Life Foods will fortify you for that mission.

Learning to Unlearn

America's #1 addiction is not cigarettes, caffeine, alcohol or marijuana. It is starches, sugar and the rest of the denatured violence we shove down our throats. William Duffy's intriguing book *Sugar Blues* rigorously explores the toll white processed sugar has taken on societies through the ages.[11] If you can do nothing else, eliminate white, unnatural sugar. This alone can begin to restore internal harmony. Witness the difference this will make in your energy level and in your moods. Like any other addict freed from substance abuse, you will be able to live a freer life.

Before you say I am ruining your life, try to stay clear of all starches for a week. Then try for a month. Retrain your mind. Reeducate your pallet

---

[11] New York: Grand Central Lifestyle. 1975.

and your digestive track. Decolonize your nutritional habits. It is to be expected that you might experience any of the following conditions; mild headaches, dizziness, an outpouring of mucus, an outbreak of acne, a discharge of hardened bile stones, a change in sleep patterns, and/or a decrease in energy. If someone complains that the Healing Crisis is gross, ask them how much grosser it is to leave fetid debris and tumors inside of you?

Fighting Back

Treat this process of destarchifying as the most intense withdrawal of your life. Expect some real initial psychological and physiological resistance. If you have ever supported or loved friends and family members as they beat heroin, oxycodone, cigarettes, alcohol, a codependent relationship or any other addiction, you know how tough withdrawal is. The withdrawal from starches and meats and dead food is no different.

To endure the starch withdrawal, it is helpful to have the support, discipline, mentorship, understanding, solidarity, guidance and love of a *Phoenix Fastician,* that is someone with experience with cleansing. We try to go through withdrawals in groups so that people have a community to rely upon. Creating a WhatsApp group can be wonderful for sharing recipes and supporting one another.

When I am fasting, I struggle at night. I often breeze through the day as a liquidarian but when the sun sets, I feel the impulse to reach for some hummus, almonds or sun-dried tomatoes with a dipping sauce (if not much more serious cheats which I won't admit here). Having a nutritional family there for you can make all the difference in the world.

Despite the challenges of what will come up, stay the course. Breathe into your transformation. This is your body letting go of toxins. This is the body going through its natural period of adjustment and recuperation. You are rebooting. Let's look at one example of how quick cleansing the liver can regenerate your health.

Tanning from the Inside Out

A Brazilian hip-hop musician and performer, Humildão, or Big Humble, became interested in Life Foods healing six years ago. Conforming to all the stereotypes of a rapper, Big Humble smoked weed all week, slept anywhere and everywhere, spilt beer on studio equipment and ate fast food on the run at scandalous, god-awful hours. He was accustomed to getting up at one in the afternoon.

When he was kicked out of his girlfriend's apartment, he came to stay on my couch. The plot thickened when he became infatuated with another girl. (No. This is not gossip. The lesson of the story is forthcoming.) Humildão became inspired to impress his new "boo" and immediately implemented radical changes. Shacked up in the Life Foods Palace in the Bronx, he took advantage of the resources that surrounded him. Humildão started training and established consistency. Within a short time, our pot-bellied, cooped-up artist was a new man. After three weeks, his long-time, underground acquaintances asked him where he was tanning and what skin products he was using. Random people commented on the inexplicable "radiance" and "brilliance" that he projected.

Humildão was light-skinned. Furthermore, it was winter. His example was illustrative. A new aura was emerging; he was a better version of himself. The most exciting part was it happened in a matter of several weeks.

The skin is a mirror of the liver and the entire digestive system. Strangers will ask Life Foodies: "Excuse me, where do you do your tanning? Nothing could be more harmful and unnatural than the radioactivity of a tanning salon. The tanning is done on the inside.

We are water. We are life. We flow like water and life. Life Foods is naturally hydrating. The circulation that gets kicked into motion by Life Foods allows for a perkier, vivacious feel and self.

This manifests itself in the hue of the skin, a spike in random smiling and in an upward surge in happy social interactions.

After destarchifying, a young woman commented: "My goodness, I just want to strike up a conversation with every cashier I come across and everyone I sit near on the train. I feel more social. I want to be me more." The most beautiful thing about this aura is that it will invite others to ask you "your secret" and hopefully emulate it so that they too can tap into their own life-vitality.

I walked into to facilitate a guest lecture at another CUNY campus and a former student suddenly emerged and hugged me. She beamed with life exclaiming "This is the professor I told you about who changed my life." I was thankful and humbled by this unforeseen introduction to the group. She shared part of her story. She talked about how she felt parts of her hips and arms that she could never feel before. I was teeming with joy for her. Her love for life was spilling out everywhere. Life Foods can work that quickly. I share this so that you too can get excited.

Liberation on a gastrointestinal level is months, weeks and even days away. For years now, I have worked with the hydro-colonics therapist, Gil Jacobs. A breatharian and liquidarian, Gil defies aging. With his school-boy grin and enviable skin,

Gil could pass as a 30-year-old. He is now well past 60. There is a Gil Jacobs locked away within all of us. It is up to us to unlock this potential that we have within.

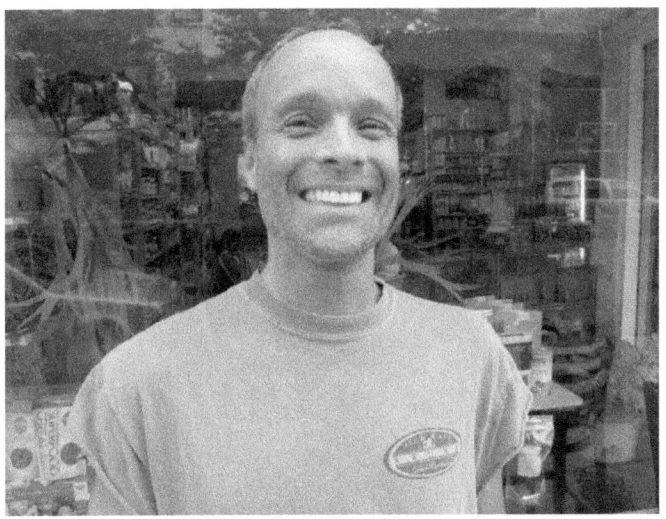

Gil Jacobs, Hydro-Colonics Therapist and eternally young

Hospitals are Sick-Houses

Krankenhaus the German word for hospital can be translated as "sick-house" or "home of the invalids." Going into a hospital is a real-life horror movie. The patients are being led around, injected with chemicals, and told when to ingest the umpteenth pill of the day. You are not on your schedule. You are on the doctors' schedule. Images that belong in a horror movie! Images that reek of death! What connection is there to nature? This is the antithesis of spirituality.

And what about the hospital food? It is mass produced. There is no individual care or affection in the preparation of the nourishment. It's comparable to prison food and school food. What does that say about those in power when our sick, our prisoners and our children are all being fed the same flimsy cardboard?

What if we could go room to room, floor to floor with a life foods dehydrator cart, teaching the sick how to heal themselves? But that will not happen under the watch of today's bloviating doctors and their overlords. Dis-ease is profit. Why would this system teach people to heal themselves if they can then forge independence from the entire system?

From the perspective of Life Foods, the sick houses are an absolute last option. Start with prevention and rebuild your immunity. Hospital patients are wild birds plucked from nature and held captive in alien cages. It is our sincerest hope that we can do everything in our power to see our loved ones free and in touch with nature. Don't let the *Krankenhaus* steal their last breaths.

The Doctor Within

The Medical Industry — which can more accurately be called The Dis-Ease Establishment — specializes in mystifying and confusing us about our suffering.

Here are a few examples. "So sorry to tell you" — the doctor says addressing my mother — "Crohn's Disease is cureless." Growing up, I was taught that strokes were like lightening; they just came out of the sky and struck down the unsuspecting, innocent victim. Parents who have obese children think it's because other people in the family are overweight. "The scientists" tell us fibroids run in our family or hemorrhoids are an inevitable, common irritation. This is pure hogwash.

A retired boxer had a blood clot. Without uttering a word about his lifestyle, the "doctors" placed metal stents in his chest, in order to reopen the veins leading to his heart. He told me his story with his head down, full of self-pity. He ended by praying for me so that "I don't suffer a similar fate."

But this wasn't fate; this was the end result of a specific lifestyle. Another close boxing friend and former opponent, Shawn McClean tragically died last year of colon cancer. He was an elite fighter and punisher but no one ever instilled within Shawn the importance of the fight within. After being diagnosed with colon cancer, the doctors at the Memorial Sloan Kettering Cancer Center put him through every form of chemo and pushed every pill on to him. Not once did they talk about any natural ways of restoring his colon. Rest in peace Shawn Mclean, a great father, fighter and friend.

As these cases show, we are all bio-individually unique and have an adverse response to toxicity. Some of us may suffer from diarrhea; others will be plagued by constipation. Some people suffer a ghastly break out of puss-filled pimples on their faces, backs or arms. Heart burn, low energy, bad breath, recurrent yeast infections, hormone concerns, acid reflux, cardiovascular issues, Irritable Bowel Syndrome, female reproductive issues and other conditions are not the result of bad luck or genetics. We are digging our own graves with our teeth, our cravings and our addictions.

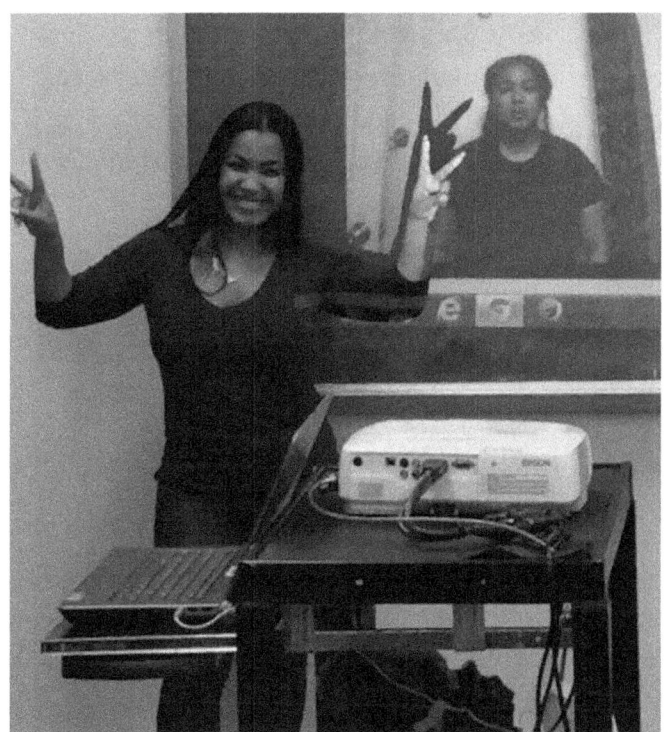

Congratulations Luzzarys -- 3 months and 60 pounds later.

There is only one Dis-ease.[12]

Our everyday lifestyle in this society has turned our intestinal terrain into a steamy bog, a veritable swamp. Our immunity is trapped in quicksand, hence unable to function as it is designed to. Our cells and digestive organs have become clogged up

---

[12] Dr. Jubb's program of cell rejuvenation is helpful in terms of its ability to begin to restore health to those who are sick. The words in quotation come from his unpublished "Phoenix Fastician Training Manual."

by the poisons we are putting into our bodies. This is called silent inflammation. The rice, the bread, the burgers, the fried food, the candy, the soda, the dairy, etc. cannot be processed and assimilated smoothly by the digestive tract.

A medical doctor worthy of their title will not just ask if you consume alcohol, smoke cigarettes or drugs. They will go deeper and inquire into how many times every week you are eating starches, sugars, meat, dairy and cooked food. It is rare that doctors ask these questions because of their own lack of training in nutritional healing.

We must start from the premise that "the body is a perfectly self-healing mechanism." Are Crohn's Disease, Irritable Bowel Syndrome and Celiac Disease real diagnosis?

These are all artificial diagnosis to keep people in the dark about their suffering. Though the diagnoses are short-sighted and misleading, the pain is all too real. The modern labels for modern problems that were brought on by modern sources of toxicity which did not exist before the Chemical Counterrevolution of the 1940's. The labels make individuals feel isolated, as though they are the unluckiest individuals on planet earth. But we are all struggling with the same dis-ease.

Another way to think about this is to consider the fact that anyone who eats gluten or strange, indigestible foods suffers from dis-ease. Because we all have bio-individuality, some responses are more extreme than others. "Doctors" offer highfalutin names so that they can swoop in atop their high horses of hubris and pretend to have cures.

We all suffer from irritable bowel syndrome and Celiac disease — gluten intolerance — on some level. Some bodies respond in more extreme ways.

The aforementioned labels for health problems distract us from the underlying problem. Treating this or that particular condition, without addressing the macrocosmic cause, may temporarily mask the anguish but it does not bring the patient any closer to healing.

Drowning and sinking in a sea of lies, how do we muster up the inner-strength to swim towards a sanctuary of self-healing?

We can heal ourselves from these conditions. This must be our starting point. We have to empower the body to do what it is designed to do.

Dr. Theodore Baroody —an acupuncturist and Certified Nutritional Consultant — wrote a book entitled *Alkalize or Die.* [13] His title says it all. Acid-

---

[13] *Alkalize or Die: Superior Health Through Proper Alkaline-Acid Balance.* North Carolina: Holographic Health Press. 1991.

forming foods — such as meats, complex carbohydrates, refined sugars and GMO's — wreak havoc on the body. Raw fruits, vegetables, sprouts, nuts and seeds have their digestive enzymes intact, providing an optimal pH balance for the body. pH is a measurement of the potential of hydrogen within a food. This determines whether a food will be able to assist the body's fluids and tissue to do their job — circulating and feeding the cells — or whether the digestive process will be stagnated.

An acidic body lacks sodium, calcium, magnesium, potassium and other essential minerals. An alkaline lifestyle neutralizes acidity. It restores balance at the cellular level and allows the body's respiratory, circulatory, and nervous system to flow optimally. We want our pH to be slightly over 7, making it alkalized. This allows for proper cellular respiration and bile flow. Bile is the liquid secreted by the liver in charge of breaking down fats to be absorbed by the body. Currently, most of us suffer from bile occlusion or bile blockages which cause all types of pain and discomfort. We need to get things flowing again. This is the function of a cleanse, to clear away debris from the arteries, liver and other digestive organs in order to free them up to do their job again. Upstream cleansing ensures that we are not polluting our sacred organs downstream.

"Ugh! My Back"

Chronic pain is horrific and prevents us from fully tapping into life's happiness.

We alter how we sit, how we sleep and our exercise patterns yet the nagging pain does not go away? Why are we a nation plagued by chronic pain?

Trapped debris is creating blockages and preventing the oxygenation of the affected area. It sounds so simple but we have to clear away the flotsam and "open up the arteries again."[14]

A Honduran doctor, Margarita was suffering from immeasurable back pain. Due to the fact that she was a doctor, Margarita thought she had tried it all. Her western (mis)-training convinced her that she was the victim of cruel tricks of nature and an unfortunate biological inheritance. She was becoming addicted to oxycodone when she began to switch up her practice. Engaging in her new-found love — a consistent yoga practice — she prodded deeper into her tissue and muscle issues.

The inflammation was not allowing her body to heal itself, resulting in acute back pain and sciatica.

After three weeks of Life Foods cleansing and her first colonics, Margarita felt a substantial amount of

---

[14] Barnard, Dr. Neal. *Food that Fights Pain*. New York: Harmony. 1999.

relief. Her pain was no longer a ☹ or a 10 on the doctors' charts. It was now a :| or a 5. Two more weeks of liquefied Life Foods cleansing and her second colonics, Margarita was moving around like a *sapito*, or little froggie. Returning to her child-like mobility, she felt light and agile. She also slept on a sleeping bag on the floor with one pillow for her head and another placed under her knees.

When she returned to work to share the good news with her colleagues, they laughed off what they saw as quackery. Enthusiastic about her new discoveries, Margarita's inner-smile saw beyond their short-sightedness. She attempted to integrate some of the natural healing into her everyday consults with patients but had to be cautious not to upset the dominant medical order.

Margarita's issue with back pain is one of the most common American ailments. The Mayo Clinic reports that there are over 3 million patients who come for relief from sciatic nerve pain every year. The good news is a combination of nutritional fasting, yoga and sleeping on the floor can help restore circulation and flexibility to afflicted areas.

Dr. Art Brownstein talks about the role stress plays in making the back muscles contract and suffer.[15] A long-time practitioner of yoga, Dr. Brownstein

[15] Brownstein, Art. *Healing Back Pain Naturally*. New York: Simon and Schuster. 2001.

teaches how the ancient school of meditation can help heal chronic pain.

Dr. Pete Egoscue's *Pain Free: A Revolutionary Method for Stopping Chronic Pain* is an excellent guide to the stretches that can help alleviate muscular-skeletal misalignment.[16] Egoscue warns against the surgical removal of pieces of the back disks and encourages a pro-active nutritional and exercise protocol, focused on rebuilding the tissue in the aggravated areas. Expounding upon the consequences of a mega-couch potato Life Style, Dr. Egoscue writes about a patient named Kevin:

"As a result of reduced oxygen, Kevin's brain, which uses about forty percent of the total oxygen intake of the body, begins to starve. It does not do so without a long struggle: Paramount as it is, the brain diverts oxygen to itself from less essential functions, running the gamut from locomotion and posture to digestion to the production of white blood cells and beyond. Meanwhile, chronic pain makes itself felt. Joints and muscles that lack oxygen cannot function properly, no matter how they are drugged, manipulated, or surgically altered. All the other systems suffer as well" (p. 25).

Dr. Egoscue advocates for natural healing because he understands that back disks and every organ in

---

[16] Egoscue, Pete. *Pain Free: A Revolutionary Method for Stopping Chronic Pain.* New York: Bantum Books. 2002.

the body are precious and have a role to play in your everyday functioning and healing. Science teaches us that the human body's capacity to heal is extraordinary; we can heal from all types of pain, discomfort and loss.

There is only one Form of Cancer — Capitalism

Every day, the American public hears about the battle against cancer. Since Richard Nixon signed the National Cancer Act in 1971, authorizing the spending of $1.5 billion on research funds over the course of three years, a "cure for cancer" has been an American obsession. We are led to believe that self-sacrificing, scientific pioneers are cooperating across the globe to find the miraculous cure. Nothing could be further from the truth.

Are we expected to believe that the most advanced and bright minds have been collaborating on finding a cure for cancer for centuries and are not one step closer to finding it? What a hoax! Instead of researching creative cures for cancer and widely publicizing the results to an anxious public, most medical professionals are part of a machinery that actively represses them. Why would the main beneficiaries of the suffering want to cure a cellular catastrophe that amounts to a \$280 billion yearly industry?[17]

The vast majority of doctors are unthinking handmaidens to the medical bureaucracy, beholden to big money. Like police officers or any other subservient bricks-in-the-wall, many doctors may be well-intentioned but they fear the consequences of challenging their superiors and losing their pay check or chances to climb up in the hierarchy. Oncologists specialize in spreading fear and demoralization. They aggressively recruit patients into dispiriting chemotherapy and radiation regiments. Introducing such hazardous chemicals to the patients' bloodstream represents a full-scale attack on their immunity. When the patients become week and pain-ridden, the doctors then prescribe oxycodone and other pain pills, further crushing the patients' will and ability to fight.

The current "War against Cancer" represents a corporate agenda. Kentucky Fried Chicken, Proctor & Gamble and other major U.S. corporations sponsor the National Breast Cancer Foundation. The pink ribbon campaign feigns concern for women in their struggle against a crippling illness but their true intent is to persuade more women to have mammograms and ensnare them in the dis-

---

[17] *The Truth about Cancer*. Part IV. This is the amount of money Americans spend every year on pharmaceutical drugs.

ease establishment. Unfortunately, for hundreds of thousands of women, early detection means early medical intervention, which all too often means early death from chemotherapy and radiation. There is evidence that mammograms themselves can contribute to causing cancer. Predictably, holistic medicine does not form part of the National Breast Cancer Foundation's agenda. Dr. Farid Fata was one doctor who was caught in the act of intentionally misdiagnosing 500 Michigan patients with cancer.[18] Chemotherapy brings billions in profits for a small coterie of elites and untold suffering for millions of our family members.

Cancer: The Monster Unveiled

Cancer is truly an American epidemic; some studies warn that one in two males and one in three women in the U.S. will develop cancer.

Cancer is presented as appearing out of thin air and striking innocent and defenseless people. This is not true. We are not powerless before cancer. The best way to wipe out cancer is to create healthy gut bacteria and never allow the malignant cells to set

---

[18] Moghe, Sonia. "Patients give horror stories as cancer doctor gets 45 years." *CNN.* July 11th, 2015.

up shop. It is wise to tackle cancer beforehand, in our teens, twenties and thirties. This will prevent the scenario of having to pick up a doctor's fear-mongering phone call, delivering the bad news and insisting we only have six months to live.

Siddhartha Mukherjee's highly-praised *The Emperor of All Maladies: A Biography of Cancer* is typical of the medical industry's treatment of cancer.[19] An oncologist himself, Mukherjee walks the reader through an exhaustive, 571-page review of every "medical breakthrough" on cancer, only to continually conclude that cancer has the upper-hand on the medical community. Having received advanced training in cancer medicine at the Dana-Farber Cancer Institute in Boston, Dr. Mukherjee remains loyal to his indoctrination and publisher, never once considering all of the scientific evidence of alternative cures to cancer. Dr. Mukherjee's book does not read as a summation of cancer-prevention research but rather as an anthology of the drug-intensive protocols adopted by the medical establishment, all of which have been a resounding failure. Typical of oncologists, not once does the "specialist" consider the myriad ways to treat cancer, such as Near Infrared Detoxing Saunas,

---

[19] Mukherjee, Siddhartha. *The Emperor of All Maladies: A Biography of Cancer*. Boston: Scribner. 2010.

Pulsating Magno-electric Field Therapy, Hyperbaric Oxygen Rooms, colonics, Gerson Therapy, coffee enemas and the full gamut of natural healing techniques with a proven track record of shrinking tumors. Turmeric, juicing, chlorophyll, oncolytic viruses, wheatgrass and hundreds of other natural remedies have also been shown to prevent and reverse cancer.[20] Incredibly, many American doctors who have dared to challenge the dominant cancer paradigm have been forced to practice medicine just south of the border in order to avoid bureaucratic FDA red tape.

Extended Life Foods Cleansing

With a proper nutritional lifestyle and the cleansing of the blood, we can beat cancer, Crohn's or any condition. By simply transforming what passes by our teeth we can repopulate our digestive tracts with healthy bacteria and rebirth ourselves in the process, tapping into unknown reservoirs of energy and healing.

Becoming a Raw Foodist is intimidating but it is doable. Change, growth and (re)birth is hard, agonizing and gut-wrenching work. Letting go of American's most common addiction will not be

---

[20] For a robust discussion of natural cures for cancer, the 9-part series, *The Truth about Cancer* is excellent.

easy. There will be infinite excuses but if we don't give our body a true shot to heal, we will never know the infinite healing potential locked within. Who has the will-power, openness and desire to take their mind body and spirit where it has never flown before? Many people — including my own family members — boast that they would rather die before they give up their vices. I fear their sarcastic wishes will be granted, long before their day has to come. We hope that they do not reach this point of no return before realizing their loved ones want to see them live longer, more vigorous lives.

The Doctors of the Future

When trying to prevent the onset of any dis-ease, such as diabetes, cancer or arthritis, as a first line of defense, you do not need medications, doctors, and hospitals. If all else fails, then there can be an open conversation, considering these extreme options.

Misinformation is everywhere. By focusing on the localized dis-ease, "the experts" never make any connections to our nutritional lifestyles. They prevent the emergence of the nutritional activist in all of us by encouraging passivity and dependency. Materialist, consumerist society has turned us into such a hapless, wretched lot. We feel sorry for ourselves. We've lost control without realizing we are self-poisoning ourselves. Yes, auto-intoxication.

Trapped financially in food deserts and stripped of empowering information, we have become the unknowing perpetrators of our own suffering.

This book has discussed why we should beware of "doctors." They almost always tell you that your condition is genetic and irreversible so that you become dependent upon them for "the cure." 40,000 new chemicals have been introduced into our foods and pharmacies in the past ten years.[21] This is a recipe for disaster.

The conventional medial response is not healing. It treats localized symptoms without addressing the underlying dis-ease. As the cover photo on this book suggests:

> *There is a pharmacy that lies within*
> *that we can tap into.*
> *This is the only pharmacy we need.*

Doctors aggressively recruit people for operations and cash in on them. Without generalizing every doctor, I have had enough of my own traumatizing experiences and witnessed others' negative experiences with doctors to see that they are poor listeners who enter into visits with patients with readymade solutions. They employ fear tactics, warning that you only have a certain amount of time to live. The critics will claim that this is an

---

[21] *Hungry for Change.* Documentary produced by Laurentine Ten Bosch and James Colquhoun. 2012.

exaggeration but this is what so many of us have lived through — hospital trauma. I can never recover what the dis-ease establishment took from me but I recovered my health and independence which they can never take from me.

As filmmaker Vikram Gandhi highlights in his brilliant documentary, *Kumaré: The True Story of a False Prophet*, there is only one shaman — the shaman within. The documentary focuses on a dozen individuals who are looking for enlightenment in Arizona and latch on to a self-anointed "guru," Vikram Gandhi himself, who is really just acting the role. What happens when they realize the truth about Vikram and his hoax?

As we undertake our journey, remember not to depend on help from outside. We are our own best alchemists. We are our own best scientists. We are the doctors of the future. There is a shaman within!

Section II. Training with Wolf[22]: Notes on a LIFE Style

As a competitive amateur boxer, with a record of 15 wins, 8 by knock out, and 5 losses, and as a yogi in training, I always want my energy to be through the roof. There are times I ran in the morning and boxed in the afternoon for three months in a row. I gallop over fields, through forests and on tracks and gollop up the miles day after day. I try to stay clear of concrete because of how unnatural it is and the damage it does on my joints and muscles over time. Some days, I do two or three workouts depending on what the universe offers. If it is a Life Water morning I might be running in the mountains taking the breaks I need to. If it is Super Bowl Sunday I might emulate Tyson Beckford's 1,500 push-ups routine or Kellin Lutz' 1,000 sit-ups challenge. I will walk you through how I organize myself to train year after year at this level of intensity.

---

[22] Lame Wolf was the name bestowed upon me by a healer trained in the Lakota tradition at the foot of the Sedona Canyons. According to the medicine man, Lame was a satirical comment on my presence before the rest of the Eagle compound. The base of the name — Wolf — denotes courage and a posture of self-defense. When I asked the good doctor if I could be Humble Wolf instead, he chuckled and said "then you would not be so humble, Wolf."

Life Foods on the Go

I pack my "granny bag" as many mornings as I can. If I have to work early, I juice the night before and have my blended smoothies and soups ready to go. Otherwise I leave a bit of prep time for the morning. In the summer, I keep a cooler in my trunk. (I know cars are not natural but our lives are replete with all types of contradictions and my son has to be in school on time.)

The Man Who Lives out of a Glass Jar

I try to prepare five or six glass jars of nutrition every time I hit the streets. I don't use plastic bottles because they leach heavy metals into our nutrition. This is called clathration. If I am going out with a group or going to a party, I might be more discreet with my nutrition or I might really flaunt it to trigger others' curiosity. My glass jars are great conversation starters. People have stared at me on the two train, in the gym or at work but when they feel the vibe and energy, they are instantly curious.

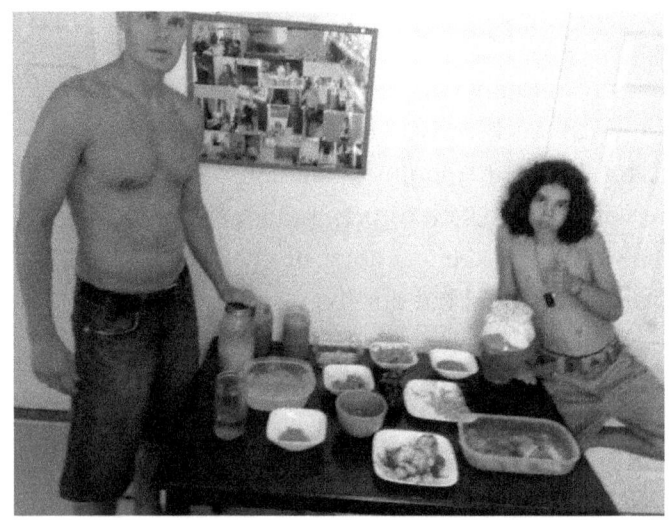

A July 4th Life Foods Buffet with Ernesto

Sleep Less, Put in More Work

Sleep is different for everybody and there are multiple variables that can impact sleep, such as stress, poor digestion and technology. From my experience during a cleanse, the shifts in my sleeping patterns are formulaic. The more I liquefy my Life Foods with the Vitamix, the more energy I have and the less I need to sleep. In contrast, a heavy, starchy meal functions as a sleeping pill because the digestive system is so overwhelmed that it robs enzymes from other parts of the body, causing fatigue. Those who constantly feel like "I have no energy," now understand why. You are over-burdening your digestive track robbing much needed energy from your muscles and brains.

Sleep is extremely important because it is when our bodies and brains reboot. A reflection of internal harmony, sleep lays the foundation for both the healthy loss and gain of weight. If you suffer from insomnia or its opposite — narcolepsy — reboot the system. There is something radically off emotionally or physiologically or both. Return to the roots. Listen to your body and ensure that you are properly rested as you undergo your journey.

If the bulk of our nourishment is blended or juiced, it is vital to learn to chew what you drink and drink what you chew. The chewing motion sets in motion digestive enzymes and activates the central nervous system to facilitate digestion. If I have writing deadlines or know that I have to produce more than extra at work on a particular week, then I will liquefy my nutrition to bolster my energy. After liquefying my meals, it is tough to go back to solids. It is like coming down off a good high. The hardest part of breaking a cleanse is ending it. The digestive system has rebooted and cannot immediately handle large quantities of food. It is important to slowly reintroduce heavier foods after a fast.

Food Journaling

What will come up and what will come out if we enter nutritional confession and dig deep to excavate our own dietary demons? Denial is a slow death. You have nothing to fear but inaction.

As you open up,
the world around you will open up
and reveal itself to you
in all of its majesty and brilliance.

Food journaling is essential in the beginning. The notebook page becomes a mirror to your gut and soul. Do you dare to take a look? Many of us have subconscious roadblocks. Documenting your lifestyle makes it more difficult to hide from it. When I go through the journals with people, they begin to stutter "Ummmmm, Ah, well actually...Like, hmmmm I may have forgotten to mention that Ah..." We cannot beat around the bush. We have to be honest with ourselves. People lie to themselves about what they eat because they feel they are getting one over on the world. But human biology leads us to the conclusion that you cannot get one over on the thyroid. You cannot fool the small intestine. You are what you eat.[23] You are the precise reflection of what has journeyed into your mouth and passed your teeth into the

---

[23] I must have heard that cliché hundreds of times growing up. It was always such a hollow saying to me. While the statement was true, I had no nutritional guidance or mentorship to elucidate what this meant. What great fortune I had to cross paths with Life Warriors at the time that I did.

esophagus. Bear down. Give your body a chance. Fight for the new you!

Victory breeds victory
Defeat breeds defeat
Food Discipline will get easier with time.

If you do not like the results of the new alkalized, fluid you, then you can always go right back to where you came from. But you will never unlock your potential, unless you try to reinvent yourself.

Barefootism and Diversifying your Training

A high percentage of runners are injured at some point of the year. I highly endorse the vibram 5-toe sneakers or better yet, *Barefootism*. Take it back to nature and your roots. Find a big baseball field, beach or park to run in. Barefoot running will tap into neglected muscles and help correct a runner's posture. Run with your hips forward, your back straight, your feet pushing off the earth, you're your glutes squeezed, like the upright soldiers, Thomas Sankara and Mamá Tingó. Barefoot jogging or sprinting sessions is like Bikram yoga in the sense that it undoes so much of the tightness we have built up in our hips, knees and lower back.

Sometimes when other people train me and implement new exercises, I feel my inner-defenses go up. Experimenting and opening up to new possibilities is challenging. The more weapons we have in our ammunition, the more prepared we are to do battle. The more flowers we cultivate, the more fragrances in our repository that we can share with the world.

I have walked into Zumba classes, pilates or salsa lessons to leave my comfort zone. How can we open up the hips? How can we tap into neglected muscles? I'm not big on weight training and the American obsession with protein but of course some weight training can be great. Most "jocks" have been socialized to make fun of what is presented here. I could have never related to nutritional transformation when I was younger.

Think of a young basketball player. They are so graceful, almost untouchable, when they soar through the air. What a high level of athleticism! But what happens to these "former" athletes as they leave their 20's. We are precipitating and accelerating our own degeneration without knowing it. We can prevent this from happening with Life Foods and maintain our athletic form well beyond our years.[24]

In their 20's, I see them Rocking

---

[24] I wrote a blog recently about a fifteen year reunion with my former teammates from the high school basketball and football teams. Time had not been kind to some of my old running mates; their deterioration was on full display.

In their 30's, I see them Scoffing
Come their 40's, they're Squawking
Come their 50's, they're flopping.

I feel the people who are most able to find Life Foods healing are those who have a real connection to nature. Being sneakerless in Van Courtland Park or Central Park for a running and yoga session, roots me back in natural training and healing. We were not born with little Air Jordans on when we zoomed out of the womb. Sneakers — while marketed as the very cure to our alignment and posture issues — may be the very cause of this problem. What is natural about $150 sneakers that elevate our heels off the ground and crowd our toes? Long distance runner Christopher McDougall's <u>Born to Run</u> makes this very argument by looking deeper into the lifestyle of the Tarahumara nation of Mexico and their ability to run extraordinary distances without injury.[25] The Tarahumara don't wear sneakers and run thousands of miles. For their traditional 100 mile collective runs through the canyons, they use home-made leather sandals. I believe correct form and the right mentality can prevent many of the injuries that plague us running addicts today. The best solution for runners' injuries is yoga, biking and swimming. We do not want to be one-dimensional athletes. I

---

[25] Random House. 2009.

just completed my first triathlon at 37, motivated by this very idea of balancing everything out.

Life Sensuality

I have done a lot of living but until I discovered the world of natural eating, I had never lived with such a heightened awareness, intense sense of purpose, and love for life. Life Force foods are addictive. When I wake up every morning, within a split second, I know what I did nutritionally the day before. I can feel it. If I broke down and had some indigestible starches, I am not at my best. I'm sluggish. I have to peel myself out of bed. I feel like I let myself down. If I have treated my body well, I feel the complete opposite. I somersault out of bed, ready to fulfill my day's work.

We cannot be overly self-judgmental when we cheat. I struggle to let go and occasionally live in the moment and have a beer with pizza or a burger. Cheating or "pigging out" for me is a major letdown. Beforehand, the anticipation is exciting and I drool when I think about sinking my teeth into a burger. In the moment, the burger — drenched in cheese, ketchup, onions and tomatoes — tastes so good. Within minutes, however, the instant gratification gives way to brain fog. I feel a food-blushing or blood-rushing into my cheeks, then into my brain. The blockages dam up the flow of my *chi.* I have said toodle-oo to part of my day because I need to take a nap so the digestive system can begin to break down these cumbersome foods.

I have had to learn this lesson many times. Now before I even cheat, I feel half excited and half disappointed in myself for even entertaining the idea. It becomes a tug of war in my mind that takes away from the enjoyment process. I am working on letting go more, not being so harsh on myself and living the moment. But the truth is that I thrive off that Life Force high. Why would I want to come down off it? When I do give in to temptation, the reality is that I produce far less, mentally and athletically.

We want this high off life feeling for our loved ones — the sensation of being at the summit of self-awareness and living life to the fullest. At family parties and reunions, how many times have we seen our loved ones hiding in the back — self-conscious — when its picture time? When it's time for a yoga class or a trip to the beach, do we sneak meekly to the back of class or hide behind our towel? When there is a high school or class reunion, how do we respond?

We want to maximize our living, not shy away from it. Explode into life.

Take up your space.
Come into your true self.

People often contact me up a few months into their transformation saying encouraging things. Brianna —who had been cleansing for only a few months — yelled into the phone: "Yeeeehaaaa! Thank you Professor Shaw! I have so much more energy." Pete, a former college soccer player, expressed: "I want to take my shirt off for the first time since college." Another young shaman in training remarked: "It's like I just want to be naked all the time." Another young brother put it this way: "Usually after having intercourse, I was done, completely tired and knocked out. Now after finishing, I am ready to go again."

Well, the juices are really flowing. You are coming into a greater mastery of your body. Does it feel good? *Yeeaah yeeaah it sure does*!

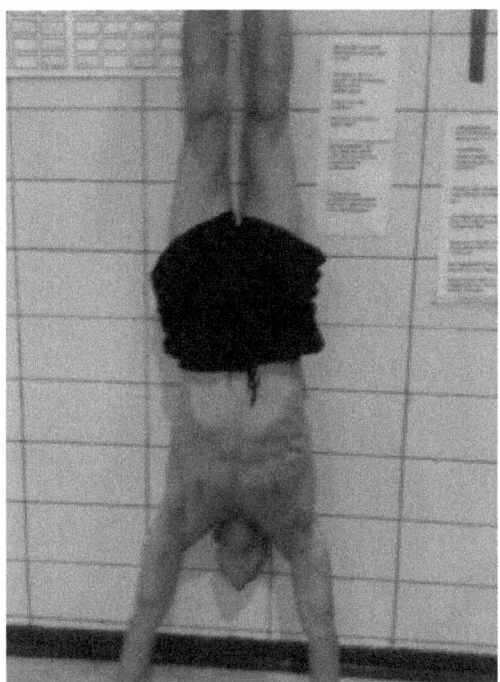

Inversions are great for blood flow and digestion.

Yoga is the perfect complement to tapping into our inner child-like vitality. Yoga makes us playful. We don't want to come out of Happy Baby and Half Pigeon. As a heavyweight fighter, I could never do somersaults and headstands. Now I strive to stand on my head or hands ten minutes a day to redirect blood flow to the neglected areas of my body. If I see my students getting lazy, daydreaming or yawning off, I'll do a quick yoga redirection of energy. Three minutes later, I can feel the difference and they can zoom back in. If only the New York City Department of Education could learn from these time-honored practices and tap into our youth's energy. Professional yes-men and bureaucrats do quite the opposite, submitting the children to overbearing test regiments and stunting their youthful vitality. When the children's' minds and bodies don't comply, they are further punished with the loss of recess, which is their only time to run free. We must take a fresh look at "hyperactivity," "autism" and "Attention Deficit Disorder." The problem is not our children; the problem is a demented world that has them and their potential penned in.

Overtraining

We should all find our favorite cardiovascular exercise and explode into it. However, there is such a thing as overtraining and it will manifest itself in a host of injuries. So be gentle and allowing. We should always train with self-love and never with self-aggression.

Sometimes the challenge is not to get the third mile but to say no to the 10th mile. I have over-trained at different times in my life. The results are never good. Coming from a family of addicts and abuse and trauma survivors, I know we all have our excesses. No question that my outlet has had its extremes.

Overtraining has manifested itself in a number of ways for me. I fought in Madison Square Garden with a hairline foot fracture. The Monday after the fight, I was on crutches. I ran too many stairs in Morningside Park, jumped too much rope, and gobbled up too many miles of concrete. I didn't have enough yoga built into my training at the time. Some winters I have felt my knees and hips screaming out for relief. Other times I have felt sharp pains in my abdomen, the middle of my chest or deep in my ribs. This was the result of taking shots in the ring and of overtraining. This is the body's natural self-preservation system sending me signals to take it easy. We have to learn to listen to the body. Having learned from the past, now I seek more balance, losing myself into two classes of yoga a day until I feel my body has been able to heal. A big part of the work I am doing today entails opening up my hips and lower back with primitive movements and yoga to undo the tightness that comes with distance running and competitive sports. Primitive movements seek to recreate the natural exercises, such as crawling and squatting, that our ancient ancestors performed in nature.

Arming yourself for the Journey

What do we need for the Life Foods journey? The Destarchifyer's kitchen should come equipped with a steamer, a Vitamix, a food processor, cheese cloths, a juicer, a dehydrator and plenty of glass jars of all sizes.   All of the recipes that follow involve these appliances. We will use the stove top burners for teas or to gently heat soups but really, we have no need for the stove. If you are working with another blender, other than the Vitamix, your smoothies will be thicker, pulpier and choppier. That is ok. The Vitamix will be by far your biggest investment at a cost of $400 to $500. But they have long warranties and are the best investment you can make for your future. If you can't get one on a credit card and pay it off, don't fret. I transitioned to Life Foods for five years, without this amazing machine and saved up $20 dollars a month in order to purchase my Vitamix. I broke 9 blenders in the process. Once I bought this machine, I could not imagine making a smoothie or homemade milk any other way. What a beauty! The Vitamix has the power to break our nutrition down to its smallest colloidal atoms. It's like pouring vitamins and minerals directly into the bloodstream.   Start building up your arsenal.

Measurements

Foods derived directly from the earth have upwards towards 1600% more nutrients and minerals than dead food.[26] Tap into the diversity of what the world provides.

Nothing in nature is measured. Nothing is boxed in or rectangular. Everything is fluid. The obsession with calorie counting leads us to false postulates. If we just focus on calories, some slices of bread may have fewer calories than a helping of macadamia nuts or almonds. But this does little to highlight the difference between calories, readily available to the body to be converted into energy, and non-deliverable calories, those which are not easily digested and get stored away in saddle-bags or love handles. I have seen too many actors, actresses, models and others obsessed with measuring everything that comes into their bodies. This is really such a self-castigating way to live. Don't limit yourself to the same measured snacks —like one apple or a couple of ounces of almonds. Liberate yourself from these suffocating expectations and structures. Tap into nature's majesty.

Many people will ask: How many meals should I eat a day?

I think we have to overthrow this entire paradigm. Sip and chew when your body calls for it. Abstain when it does not. Learn to listen to the body. There

---

[26] Dr. David Jubb. 2006. *The Phoenix Fastician Manual.* Unpublished.

are days I don't have any proper meals in the traditional sense. I sip Mango Electrolyte Lemonade by morning, teas by afternoon and a blended soup and nut milk by night. While this appears impossible in the beginning, it soon becomes natural as we retrain the mind and body and decolonize the taste buds. There are other days and occasions that call for a bona fide Life Foods banquet. If I have company I might prepare a hearty quinergy-based crust and dehydrate some zucchini bread with Life Burgers or fire up an all-you-can-eat Life Foods Pizza and Pasta night. It's all flowing. It's all contingent on the moment and what is called for.

There is no need to call me up at 2 a.m. to report that the spinach bisque was better with 2 cups of water rather than 1 1/2. Nothing is set in stone. Don't suggest how a recipe might taste for others. I don't like naming my dishes or telling people what is inside of them until they have partaken in the glory. Suggesting takes away from their trek through nature. Let them find out for themselves. We all have bio-individually unique taste buds and needs. Build up your confidence by training in the Life Foods kitchen with others and experimenting. If something is radically off, radically readjust it. The truth is not on the sidelines but in the trenches of personal and collective transformation. Only you can forge your own path and define what nutritional program works for you.

Breathing into Your Hunger

Though this might sound insane, at times it is good to sit with and breathe into your hunger. Ask yourself is this emotional hunger or physiological hunger? I try to follow this mantra: Never eat when you are angry. Never eat when you are stressed. Never eat when you are sad. Never eat when you are in a hurry.

I taught *Understanding Cultural Diversity* at York College in Jamaica, Queens, NYC for the past 7 years. I taught night time courses. It was a long commute on the train from the Bronx. I noticed if the administration was breathing down my neck about the curriculum or if something was off emotionally when I hit the E train, I was just fuming. The rage made me want to say "Forget all this" and grab a falafel or a Jamaican veggie patty. From the perspective of some readers, that may appear to be a healthy decision. It's all relative. Yes, it's better than *Murder King, Crackdonalds* or *Blubway* but the falafels and patties are fried and processed. We don't want them in our precious bodies. The point is that the emotional tension was looking for an outlet and food is among the most immediately gratifying pleasures on earth.

When I feel emotional hunger, I try to retreat into yoga, breathing or meditation. I explore my breath and accept that depression, anger, fear, disappointment and abandonment are human emotions to be experienced and embraced, not treated with synthetic chemicals.[27]

Go deeper into your emotions. The mind and body are intimately connected. One cannot be at peace if the other is not. Upon arising from the breathing exercise, I whip up a nice juice or tea to see if that settles my stomach. Then I can evaluate what my body truly needs in terms of honest nourishment.

Stylizing the Life Foods Kitchen

The gut is the center of our individual universe. All dis-ease and all healing are generated there. The Life Foods kitchen is the workshop where we heal the gut and reinvent ourselves.

When people ask me my favorite restaurant I say "The Life Foods Palace." They reply "Oh wow, I never heard of it. Where is that? Wait isn't that your address?" Of course, there are times to be

---

[27] For more reading on the emotional side of things I recommend Pema Chodron's *When Things Fall Apart*. I call it the break up book because it teaches us that we must let go of expectations and the need to control things. Everything in life is temporary and uncertain. Breathe into the transient, impermanence of it all.

social and to partake in collective merriment and feast. We do not want to come across as cultish hermits. In general, however, I try to prepare my foods at home before I set out for the day. Yes, it is a great deal of preparation time but your body will be infinitely grateful.

The reader can imagine how close friends burst into laughter when I show up somewhere with my army of glass bottles covering the entire spectrum of colors found in nature. It's all balance.

Our kitchens should exude life. Decorate your sanctuary with pictures and scents that inspire. Clear the way. Unclutter. Organize everything. My teas are on this shelf. My spice game is over here. I have an array of oils — coconut oil, flax seed, avocado, walnut, olive oil etc. — on this shelf. I dispose of cereal, rice, legumes and canned goods or at least segregate them to the furthest confines of my kitchen, to lessen the temptation. I put my fruit basket in the center of the kitchen table. There are windows open and flowers in full bloom. There is a kaleidoscope of colors that draw the visitor in.

A cluttered kitchen is a cluttered bloodstream. Just as we sweep the intestinal tract clean, we must sweep away the debris on the kitchen floor.

Before we can take a cuuc to the huum[28]

---

[28] A cucumber dipped in hummus.

we must take a mop to the floor.

Take great pride in your kitchen. This is the center of your home and of your entire being. If there is no order here, how can we have order elsewhere? When I am leading people through a cleanse, the first thing I do is clean out their cupboards and give the refrigerator a makeover, scrubbing and scraping away debris. Sometimes it's good to go in with an army of volunteers especially if someone's kitchen is in severe neglect and old potatoes are transmuting into vodka atop the stove, as I have observed before.

I separate Life Foods from Death Foods in the cabinets. In the beginning the Life Foods section of the kitchen may be minimal. You may only have a carton of almond milk, some berries, raw honey and coconut oil. That is the first step. You are invested in a new you. But you have to be the one to actually deposit the refuse where it belongs. I cannot throw it away or donate it to a shelter for you.

Building a Life Foods Body

Life foods unto itself will not give you muscle tone and definition but it will optimally position you to do so. What appears to be a lifestyle of self-deprivation is in actuality a nutritional feast. The clearing away you have done positions the body to absorb a maximum amount of minerals.

If it was easy,
It just wouldn't feel right.

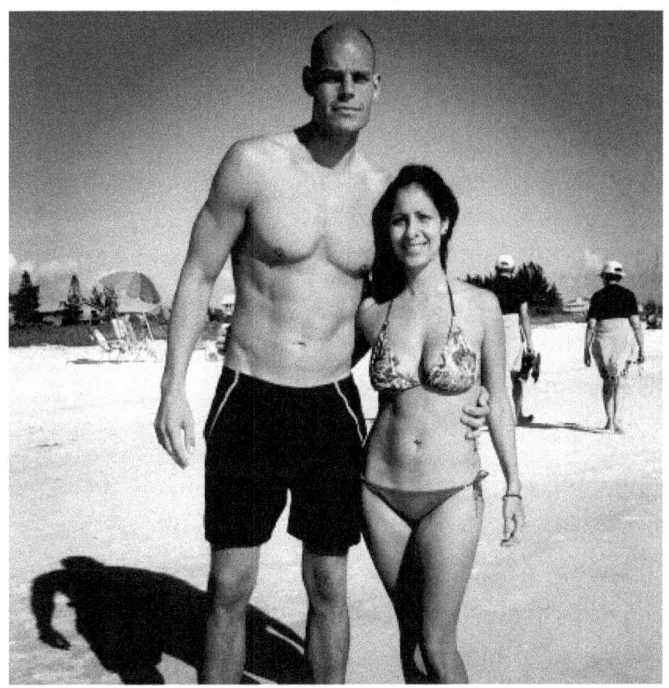

Hard work!

The body itself can produce up to 15 grams of protein as well as many amino acids and minerals that we need to thrive. The problem is that we are unintentionally preventing our bodies from doing what they are capable of doing, by overburdening them. Unlock the potential.

A former college running back #39 lost 39 lbs. in the course of 6 months on Life Foods. #39, Vinny, was very disciplined. The discipline he learned on the football field, in the weight room and in the class room was now applied to Life Foods.

The results were astounding. He repeatedly expressed that he felt so alive but also felt "skinny." He had indeed slimmed down. Goji berries and maca powder, unto themselves, will not "cut" you up. There is no substitute for hard work. You have to ask yourself: did you do 100 push-ups and sit ups in the morning and the afternoon? Can you work towards 1000? How many runs did you get this week? Beyond yoga, he had not been pushing himself.

Vinny's Phase II was to return to running, drills, sprint work and strength exercises he had not revisited in sixteen years. The old running back was back! Instead of reminiscing about his glory days like Al Bundy, he had many more glory days to live. He adopted the following slogan to capture his new lifestyle:

"From Chuggin 40's to Runnin' 40's"

There can be no doubt that we can reverse the aging process. Lifefoodarians don't get older. We youth! We don't die. We multiply. The goal is to be:

Quicker and lighter at 40 than at 20.

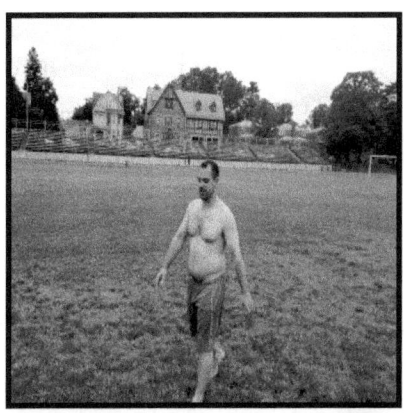

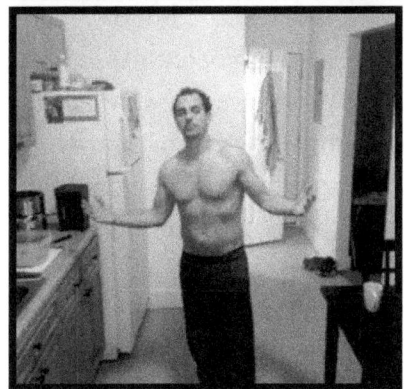

Vinny, #39: toned up and ready to go.

Good Going #39!
You have found the hidden
and forbidden fountain of youth.
You have chosen to be a spring chicken for life.
We reversed the aging process.
We are real life Benjamin Buttons.

Measuring someone's "age" by a number tells us nothing about their lifestyle. When people ask me my age I offer up some smart-aleck answers. I'll simply state that I am a lot younger than I was seven years ago. Or I'll say I'm two, explaining that I transcended my first lifetime of self-inflicted slow death and emerged into a new lifetime of healing.

The Ego: How am I Supposed to Look?

This society misconstrues protein, strength and how we "should" look. Our natural builds — freed from all of the puffed-up, bloated-ness induced by starches and GMO's — are leaner than we tend to imagine. This allows for a maximum range of motion and a return to child-like mobility. For a society constantly striving for *Bigger, Stronger, Faster*, as evidenced in the 2008 documentary about the abuse of steroids in sports, Life Foodarians can inevitably appear "too skinny."[29] My old boxing world and family constantly judge my lifestyle. They are suffering from a myriad of curable illnesses, yet they label people who set out of the box as "weird." They lurch from one medication and doctor's appointment to the next but insist on judging others who disrupt this routine. Something does not add up. I love them and fear for them. I

---

[29] *Bigger, Strong, Faster.* Directed by Christopher Bell. 2008. Documentary.

hope their psychic and gastro-intestinal discomfort turn into real changes.

Life Foods provides for a leaner, athletic definition. I fought in Madison Square Garden twice at 235 pounds. When I am on top of my game, I walk around today at 210 pounds. I feel like this is my natural Life Foods, destarchifyed weight. After months of disciplined training and work, I can come down to 195 lbs.

Though the outside world may misconstrue me at 195, seeing me as weak and frail, I knew spiritually that this was my emancipated self. I was lighter, sharper and more inefficient in all facets of my life. The god-size, judgmental gaze from my family and community did not align with how I was feeling. Letting go of expectations and pleasing others, I tapped deeper into my own internal fortitude. Less weight equals less baggage. Your self-emancipation is right around the corner.

Many men have been socialized to equate big muscles with masculinity. The female version of this comes in the form of "yes I want to train but I don't want to lose my curves." That is understandable but can you go deeper? Our unique anatomies are to be embraced. However, excess weight — whether it is in tummy, derriere, boobs or thighs — holds parasites and is unhealthy. Do what you do because it makes you feel great, not because it pleases anyone else.

Defining the right weight for ourselves is an internal struggle we all have to go through. There is an ongoing war against our self-images and self-esteem. Pursue your goals, relentlessly, but learn to love yourself in the process. This can sometimes be the toughest part. There are enough external forces (i.e. heterosexism, the pornography

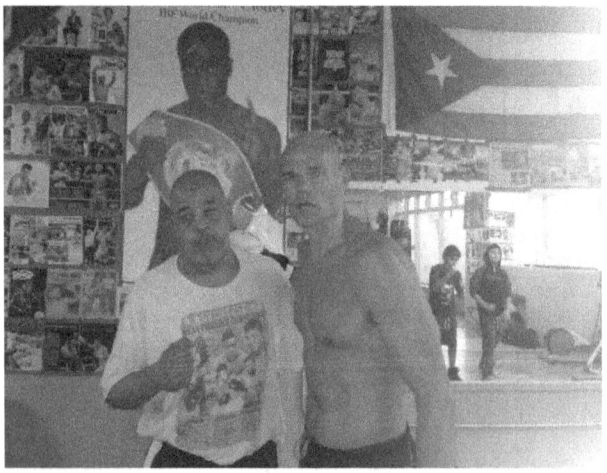

No longer a heavy weight fighter, with my trainer, the Cuban Lazzaro Almanzar

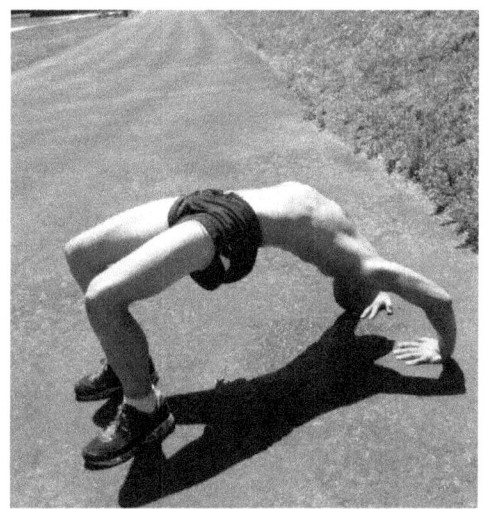

In bridge pose, 45 pounds lighter than when I was a heavy weight

industry, misogyny, machismo, the advertising industry, the evening news, etc.) trying to cut us down. We have to build up an internal fortress of healing and self-love. Don't let any outside force define your happiness; only you yourself can define it!

Radical Acceptance

According to the American Society of Plastic Surgeons, in 2015, there were 15.9 million plastic surgeries.[30] Compared to the year 2000, breast lifts are up 89% and buttock lifts are up 252%. This

---

[30] American Society of Plastic Surgeons. "Annual Plastic Surgery Statistics Reflect the Changing Face of Plastic Surgery." *Science Daily.* February 25th, 2016.

translated into a buttocks implant every 30 minutes in 2015. The Society lamented that the number of patients were "so low."

For the first time, men accounted for 40% of breast reduction surgeries, indicating the nefarious effect of the SAD die-t on men's figures.

With plastic surgery normalized, are we becoming the first generation of mutants?

We still don't know what the ramifications of the foreign silicone implants and tummy tucks. It may take another twenty years before the research exists to calculate just how invasive and harmful plastic surgery is. The effects of Botox and these foreign chemicals have never been tested on the body. Gastric bypasses unnaturally mutilate the gut and disarm it from doing what it is designed to do.

There are horrific cases of death that have resulted from too much anesthesia and severe blood clotting during these gruesome surgeries. Four years ago, we lost a colleague who went to have a clandestine operation done in the Dominican Republic.

The decision to alter one's body is surely one's own decision. Who I am to judge anyone's personal motivations?

The penetrating question, from a sociological angle, is why can fewer and fewer of us accept our natural figures? What is it in the superstructure (TV, advertising, radio stations, etc.) of society that is influencing more young people to radically alter their nature-given bodies? How can we learn to accept and love ourselves more with all of our nature-given diversity?

Succumbing to the belief that surgery is a magic bullet to all of their problems, most patients don't change their lifestyle. In real life, there are no easy shortcuts to healing. Remember: the doctor is within.

From Sexual Exploitation to Partnership

The nutritional trek is never detached from never-ending spiritual growth in other areas of our lives. Forging healthy sexuality is an important part of this growth.

I was walking down 149th St. past 3rd Ave. in the Bronx on the first day of summer. A woman with bleach blond hair strolled down the avenue. What transpired was like a scene from a movie — every group of men she passed by ceased all of their activity to stop, stare at her and yell lewd comments at her.

I took a road trip to the beach last summer with four friends that came together from different social circles in my life. There was a boxer, a vegetarian, a community organizer and my cousin.

The two-hour drive sounded like a chest-beating macho-contest. The crew traded stories about how many girls they were with and how hard "they gave it to them."

It sounded like every rap song that is promoted by the mainstream media. Women were sexual objects to be "banged, nailed etc."

My nutritional voyage has been aligned to another spiritual journey, that of transcending many of the unhealthy habits and attitudes I had learned to have towards women.

Through this process of redefining what we eat and how we see the world, our self-image, and our expectations about weight and image, we grow beyond the limits imposed on us. As we learn to open up to the world, the world unfurls itself to us, with all of its infinite grace and majesty.

We learn to be more gentle and vulnerable, more honest and loving. We, men, hiding behind a veneer of masculinity and invincibility, learn to tear the veil off.

It is not us. We've been so busy living for others, we lost sight of our own internal child. We are afraid to feel, to express, to be intimate and vulnerable.

Patriarchal, white supremacist society has conditioned us men in violent, anti-women ways.

We have learned to see women not as our spiritual and intellectual equals but as possessions — to be used, flaunted and discarded.

There's a thin line between lust and disgust in the mind of men, conditioned and trapped in a heartless, patriarchal work.

Tantric yoga and love-making can cultivate a deeper bond with your partner. Through the practice of Karezza, the goal shifts from an individualist climax to the building of trust and partnership.

In the words of Dr. Bernard Jensen, author of *Love, Sex and Nutrition*, "To attain the most exalted state of happiness and fulfillment, it is necessary to help someone else get there, too."[31]

There is also an abundance of research that as a society we men are "over-ejaculating," causing signification damage to our prostates and testes. Celibacy and tantric love-making can help individuals and couples transcend much of the poison we have internalized as products of this

---

[31] *Love, Sex and Nutrition: A Nutritional Guide to Improving and Energizing Your Intimate Relationship.* New York: Penguin Group: 1988.

violent society.[32] What is abstinence but another form of fasting, a spiritual fast that is very important for our growth as healthier fathers and men?

There are powerful fellowships such as SAA and SLAA, composed of men and women focused on forging this healthy sexuality. The struggle against the patriarchy we have internalized is a constant and necessary one.

What if God smoked Cannabis?

Ganja is big in nutritional circles. I never had a relationship with marijuana. This was one of the reasons I was motivated to write this book and tell my story. I was unique from the small Life Foodist circle around Dr. Jubb. I worked full time and I was an athlete. This was something that was disappointing to me about some of the Life Foodarians who trained me in the kitchen. Some had fallen into a lazy, sedentary lifestyle. As they ruminated on how to "seize the banks and control the money supply," they chain-smoked marijuana and organic tobacco. I wasn't looking for a washed up, burnt-out hippie scene; I was looking for motivated, well-grounded and pro-active nutritionists.

---

[32] Research Gil Jacobs on YouTube for more information on this topic.

I don't believe in any form of smoking. This is not a moral view but rather a nutritional assessment. Of course, if done under the right spiritual guidance, there can be a time for this but in general smoking is very harsh on the throat, esophagus and lungs. Smoking tar creates carcinogens. One my mentors, Steve Melken of Chefchaouen, Morocco, was a Raw Foodist for 40 years, but still died of throat cancer. From what Raw Foods Steve could gather, as he fought until the very end, was that years of smoking organic, homegrown marijuana from the mountains of north Morocco, took its toll on his body.

Smoking does not form part of my lifestyle. If the reader was so inclined to dabble in the herbs, it is better to ingest it through an enjoyable Life Foods mix, such as cacao, coconut oil and sunflower lecithin. The use of marijuana can be great for natural, non-addictive pain management and for bolstering the appetite. Eating it is much easier on the body in the long term and provides for a nice whole-body high. Soak your trees for two weeks in coconut oil before trying this at home. You can also establish a nice little paste with coconut oil, carob, and some blended fruits. Take off from there!

Section III. The Destarchifyer's Foundation:

Life Foods Recipes

I have organized the recipe booklet in the order in which I integrated these life-affirming foods and drinks into my life. I start with the easiest recipes to learn and move towards that which are more time-intensive. It is worth experimenting with everything and then seeing what balance works best for you. Every recipe is a mystery until it is broken down to its components and you prepare it yourself. We don't learn through reading but rather by practicing in the Life Foods kitchen. You may find my measurements to be too much or too little. Make those adjustments as you see fit. Remember you can always add but you can't subtract.

Often when we begin cleansing, we eat lots of salads and smoothies because that is what we are most familiar with. This simplicity can begin to weigh on you after a while. The more diversity you bring to your pallet, the more prepared you will be for the journey.

I have included 32 recipes, with notes on how to tweak them in different ways. There are dozens or other concoctions that I utilize and discover constantly. By studying and adopting this lifestyle, infinite options will present themselves allowing you to build upon your repertoire. It is akin to experimenting with different compounds in chemistry. Many of these suggestions are recipes for a recipe. In other words, once you learn the art of making a blended soup, a smoothie, kombucha, a life bar, a fresh juice or a dehydrated burger or meatloaf you can make up your own.[33] There is no right or wrong. Your taste buds should be in command.

It is worth remembering that liquefying your nutrition through the Vitamix is the most powerful and efficient way to deliver nutrition to your cells. Aim to be a liquidarian when you can. I assure you the results will be nothing less than amazing and this will move you in the direction of occasional breatherianism. Breatherianism involves fasting entirely and deriving energy from alternative sources, such as the sun and breathing.

---

[33] Does calling something a burger necessitate that it has flesh? What are burgers, dogs, breads and cheeses but paradigms waiting to be undone and reinvented? What masters of taxonomy decided what constitutes a burger? We want burgers, buns and biscuits that have both good taste and offer up good energy.

Cherry Electrolyte Lemonade

Great for cleansing the digestive tract and giving it a much-needed rest! The easiest Life Foods on the go. A foundation for the Liver and Gall Bladder flush. Use this to get you through the a.m.

3 organic lemons
  (Cut off the skin, white pith included, organic better of course.)
1 apple or pear cut up
  (Get creative with cherries, mangos, strawberries etc.)
4-5 tablespoons raw honey (adjust for sweetness)
2 tablespoons coconut oil or try flax seed oil, olive oil, almond oil etc.
A pinch of Celtic sea salt for hydration
5-6 cups filtered or charged water, or more depending on your taste buds
Blend all ingredients in a Vitamix (If you don't have a one, you might have to juice the lemons with the skin. Or blend and then strain)

Life Foods on the Go — Snacking

Here are some really simple tricks when you are caught in a bind, working and racing around in the concrete jungle or you if you are in the hippie van road-tripping.

- Grab some Brazil nuts or pecans and wrap them up in sun dried tomatoes.
- Get some nori sheets and dip them in hummus.[34] Always have a freshly brewed tea or kombucha packed with chia seeds wherever you go. This is good to stave the appetite and settle the stomach. Carry some goji berries, dried mango and watermelon with seeds.
- Watermelon is of course amazing. Mix it up by sprinkling some Celtic sea salt on yours.
- Trail mixes are yummy. Just make sure there are no peanuts or anything processed, heated or coated with sugar in your trail mixes.
- Local health food stores — while expensive — have some good combos. The sprouted chia cacao or ginger buckwheat cereals are excellent snacks as well with or without your nut milk.

---

[34] Hummus is not a Life Foods. Chick peas are a legume which can be a bit heavy on the digestive track. Stay clear of canola oil and soy bean oil. There is also a homemade Brazil nut hummus we can integrate into our regiment.

- Never think of this as Die-ting. You are adding. You are opening up the spectrum. There is no deprivation. On the contrary, there is a magnifying of possibilities.

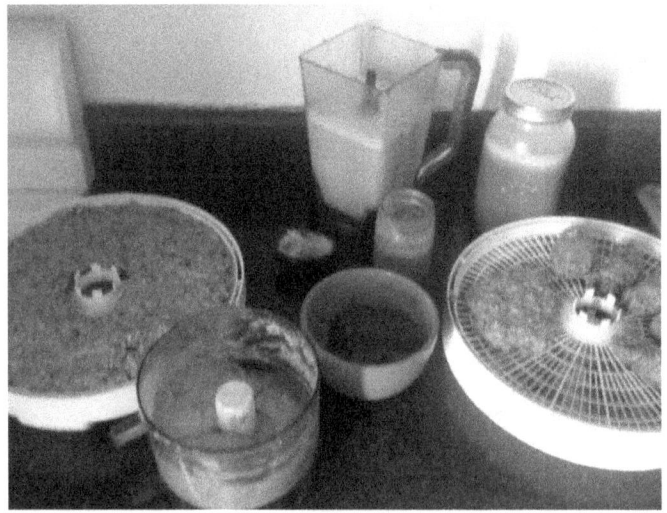

Morning prep! Getting ready to hit the streets

Collard Greens with Tahini Sauce

(You can substitute broccoli, spinach, chard, kale, bok-choy, etc. but steam for less time.)

Onwards to the Steamed Promise Land
Lightly steaming our vegetables does not kill off its life force. As long as temperatures do not exceed 117 degrees, we have upheld life and have no blood on our hands.

- Steam collard greens (try 10 minutes or a few more)
- Steam sliced white or red onion with red pepper for 5 minutes
- 3 tablespoons tahini hummus (a non-zionist brand of course)
- Sprinkle Celtic sea salt in the different layers of greens
- Add a few squirts of Braggs amino acids
- Sprinkle with pecans, walnuts or almonds
- Sprinkle sliced dried mangos, apricots or cranberries
- Mix everything together for an absolutely lovely, filling dish.
- Then try a tbsp. of turmeric, Apple Cider Vinegar, Italian seasoning, Lemon pepper, basil, cayenne pepper, oregano, cumin or any combo…The spice game is infinite.

Ginger Plum Sauce

Try this sauce with the steamed veggies:
1/4 cup Almond Butter
1-2 cloves garlic
3 tbsp. Raw Tahini
Few tbsp. Braggs Amino Acids
1 plum
1 tbsp. raw honey
1 tbsp. apple cider vinegar
¼ of lemon squeezed for juice
½ piece of ginger
1 tbsp. olive oil

Pure Juicing Ingenuity

Buy a Vitamix before you invest in a juicer, if that is possible. Blending is superior to juicing. This is not in question. Many of the nutrients are in the seeds and skin of fruit. We don't want to lose any of the fiber. But I still believe juicing has a place in our everyday efforts, if for nothing else to give variety to what we do. I find the juicer to be very helpful when flavoring my kombucha or preparing my electrolyte lemonades. My cellular energy is off the wall when I juice, so I still integrate this into my life! But yes you are losing some of the nutrients such as vitamin U, a powerful enzyme. Juice the following

- Sour green apples, sweet red apples, grapes, ginger, lemons, limes, cucumber, celery (penetrating and acrid, not my favorite but very good for sexual energy), pears, and melons.
- The most powerful greens such as spinach: kale, dandelion and lamb's quarters.
- Peaches and plums.
- Try garlic. Good for the heart.
- Mix and match to your heart's delight. You will never get bored.
- The toughest thing about juicing is the cleanup. It can be time consuming. So make it in bulk. Have a few liters at your

disposal. Keep them in glass jars so the plastic is not bleeding into your purity.

- Throw straight vitamin C in there for more of a boost but this can offset the taste some.
- To have even more endurance use the Tarahumara nation's secret, Chia Seeds *(soak in the juice for 15 minutes, give it a shake and you are ready to go.*

Lift off! — Stay High off Life like Fred Hampton — Soar and See what was once Unseeable.

The Alkaline Kidney Replenisher

- Juice cucumber
- parsley
- celery
- kale
- berries
- lemon
- Add vitamin C and some high alkaline water to taste.

Kombuchando Recipe

For thousands of years, the Chinese have used this fermentation to prevent cancer and the onset of other illnesses. As you get your routine down, invest in larger glass bottles to expand your operations.

Every batch of kombucha is unique. You'll pick up your own rhythm through trial and error. The first step is to get a scoby aka the kombucha mushroom culture. Anyone who is fermenting their own kombucha can get you started.

(This is for a 7-cup glass bottle.)

- Make sure the utensils, hands and pot are clean.
- Boil 1 liter (4 cups) of water for 5 minutes then turn off the stove.
- Add 4 or 5 bags of tea. Try ginger lemon, green tea or mango peach tea. This will color and flavor the batch.
- Add (1 ½ cups) of regular white sugar or 6 big scoops of raw honey. The kombucha will feed and grow off this but this will not enter into your bloodstream by the time the brew is ready. Stir the hot water and sugar so that it dissolves.

- Add 5 cups of filtered water. This water will quicken the time for the tea and sugar brew to cool down.
- Add the sugar and tea water into the jar with water.
- Let this cool down. Any heat will kill the scoby. The jar should just feel cool or no more than 98 degrees.
- Put in the starter brew approximately 2 cups plus 60 ml (1/4 cup) of Apple Cider Vinegar. (The vinegar helps the fermentation process. The sweetening agent provides carbonation. So, more sugar more carbonation.)
- Add the scoby with the brown bits (the yeast) face down.
- Cover jar with paper towel and a rubber band around the neck.
- I have my kombucha empire in a closet where I can easily move them in and out every week when I start a new batch.
- By day 14 or 20, check the brew and it should be carbonated and fermented. Depending on your taste, you can put into glass bottles with sliced berries or any fruits and let the glass bottles sit for further fermentation. After 2 weeks, you should have super fizzed out booch.

- Save 2 cups as the starter brew for your next batch. Make another batch as soon as you begin drinking the new batch.
- You will notice the first couple of batches may be weaker in taste and carbonation but the 3rd batch on gets really fizzy.

Kombucha Kings Exclusive

Here are some flavors to experiment with in your glass jars, once your kombucha has brewed for a few weeks. Cut them up and put into the smaller jars. Wait 2 weeks then discard the fruit and enjoy your kombucha.

- Dried fruits: apricot, goji berries
- Grapes, pineapple, strawberry, apples, berries, pear, cranberries (juicing or blend and strain)
- Ginger, lemon
- Super food, green powder, spirulina
- Coconut sugar, turmeric.

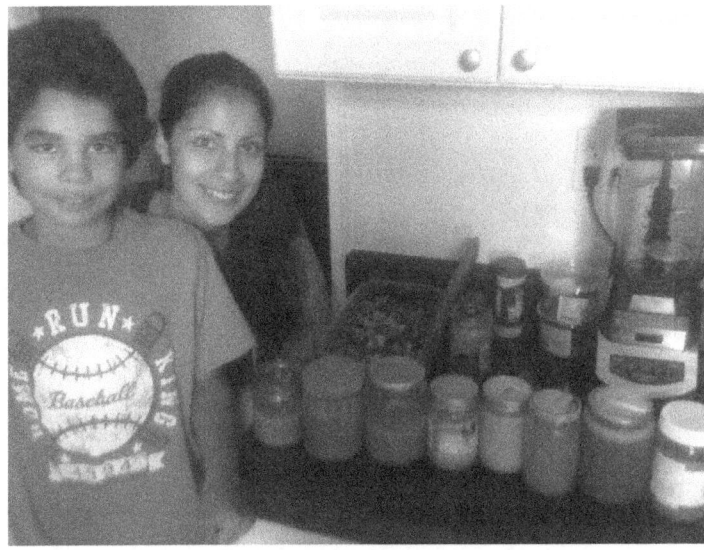

Kombucha for a Road Trip

The Aura of the Amazon

- Pack of Açaí
- Half a bag of frozen mangos (or peaches or try frozen butter nut squash too)
- 10 cherries
- Half a banana
- 1 tbsp raw honey
- 1 tbsp coconut oil
- 1.5-2.5 cups of water depending on how thick you want it

The Eternal Inca Bomb-Berry Smoothie

- 4 cups of almond milk
- Heaping teaspoon of chocolate hemp protein
- Heaping teaspoon of sunflower lecithin
- Heaping teaspoon Monk fruit sweetener
- Fistful of Andean gooseberries
- Heaping tablespoon of Incan Lucuma powder
- Fistful of frozen butternut squash
- 1 banana
- small helping of Irish moss

Enjoy and Live Forever!

Life Foods Lime Margarita Mix

Blend the following in the vita mix

- 2 cups of cherries
- 2 peeled limes
- 1 green apple cut up
- a heaping tbsp. of raw honey
- 1/2 tbsp. of coconut oil
- 6 cups of water

Chichi's Fresh off the Boat Watermelon Float[35]

- Blend ¼ of a watermelon
- Juice or Squeeze 2 or 3 lemons or limes
- Two ice cubes
- 2 tsps. raw honey
- Pinch Celtic sea salt
- Some high alkaline water to get it to blend.

Voila a very nourishing, water-rich picker-upper. Once you have tried that, bring in spoonfuls of cherries, mango or cantaloupe to switch up the taste. This is very good on hot days or after a workout any time of the year.

---

[35] I named this one after my son Ernesto because he was there with me and we developed it together. His nickname, "Chichi" means baby in the Dominican Republic. And how truly beautiful to train a young mind in the kitchen! They will always have an option that many of us never had access to.

Macadamia Nut Vanilla Ice Cream

The Watermelon Float is amazing unto itself or you can make a homemade Vanilla float as well.

- Blend up 1 cup macadamia nuts (*They are extremely overpriced at $19.99/lb. If you have a cute 9-year-old, you can sneak some into his pockets. Just don't get caught. It can be quite embarrassing or much worse.*)
- 1/5 cup of soaked and thoroughly cleaned Irish Moss (*and then increase if you enjoy it*)
- 2 tbs. Raw honey
- 2 tbs. alcohol free Vanilla extract
- ¼ to ½ tbsp. Celtic sea salt
- ¼ cup Almond, walnut or Brazil nut milk

The No Compromise Green Monster

- 1 pack of Acai
- 2 slices of Mamey
- 2 chunks of Watermelon
- 1 handful of Gogi berries
- 3 cups Almond milk
- A Pinch Celtic sea salt
- 1 scoop raw Cacao
- 1 scoop Chocolate Hemp Protein
- Handful of Spinach
- 5 Macadamia nuts
- 2 tbsp. Bee pollen
- 2 tbsp. Raw honey
- 2 tbsp. Coconut oil or Almond oil
- 1 tbsp. Sunflower Lecithin
- 2 ice cubes
- Vita-mix it up!

Red Owl's Fiery Broth

Blended soups are very important in Life Foods. They are hearty but light. If you are "starving," prepare a blended soup before you indulge in other temptations.

- Begin with the Emulsification of 3 tbsp. oil, 2 tbsp. lecithin, 1 tbsp. raw honey, and ½ tbsp. Celtic sea salt
- 2 Garlic cloves
- 1 small white Onion
- 4 pieces of Celery
- 1 tbsp. Black pepper
- 1 tbsp. Turmeric
- ½ tbsp. lemon
- Small piece of ginger
- 1 tbsp. Jerk seasoning (more for spiciness)
- 2 tbsp. Chia seeds
- Blend in a Vitamix and heat to your desire.
- Slice and lightly steam any combination of mushrooms, cabbage, spinach, squash, and or asparagus. Pour the steamed vegetables into the now heated broth for a filling soup.

Teofilo Stevenson
Blended Spinach Bisque

- 2 cups spinach
- Small white onion steamed
- Red pepper steamed
- Steam for 5 minutes.
- Then put in the blender with the following
- 3 garlic cloves
- 2 massive tbsp. of miso
- Piece of ginger peeled
- 1 massive tsp nutritional yeast
- 1 Tbsp. raw tahini
- ¼ tsp Celtic sea salt
- ¼ cup cold-pressed Olive Oil
- 2 tbsp. parsley[36]
- 2 tbsp. oregano
- 3 basil leaves
- ½ cucumber
- ½ turmeric powder
- 3 tbsp. Bragg's Liquid Amino Acids
- 2-2 ½ cups filtered water
- (Add a little hot chili pepper or cayenne if you want to go the spicy route)

---

[36] I measure in tablespoons but fresh sprigs are of course so much better for us.

There's nothing to it but to do it. Experiment and perfect the taste for your pallet.

This is a basic Life foods soup recipe. You can then substitute steamed butter nut squash, cauliflower with red pepper or other veggies. You can make adjustments. Be inventive. If you are missing one ingredient, substitute it with another.

Blended Sun-Dried Tomato Soup

Piquant and Provocative

- Soak 1 cup of sun dried tomatoes for 15 minutes
- 1 cup of Brazil or Almond nut milk (*heat with the water but don't bring to boil, a good test of the heat is if your pinky can wade freely in the water*)
- 1/2 cup filtered water
- 1/4 cup Irish moss (*soaked for 2 days and thoroughly cleaned*)
- 2 tbsp. Italian seasoning
- 2 tbsp. oregano
- 4-6 vine tomatoes (*smaller ones*)
- 1-2 cloves of garlic (*or more to taste*)
- ½ tsp of Celtic Sea salt or more but remember you can always add you can't take away
- ½ tbsp. lemon juice fresh squeezed
- 1/8 - 1/4 cup of Olive Oil
- ¼ cup nutritional yeast
- 1/2 tbsp. turmeric
- Optional pinch of cayenne or some jalapeño
- Blend all this then bring in the sun-dried tomatoes and Re-blend.

Once you have confidence with this recipe, you can get playful with your soups. Do I want to blend in some sweetness? Maybe 5 soaked apricots. Maybe a piece of avocado for some creaminess? Maybe some macadamia nuts for thickness? There are no limits. "At the top, it's just us."

Un-sautéed Arugula & Mushroom Magic

- Steam mushrooms, garlic and onions for 8 minutes
- bring arugula in for the last 2 minutes
- season with
- sweet peppers
- tomatoes
- a dash of jalapeños
- a dash of lemon
- tbsp. tahini
- tbsp. coconut oil (or more if you are feeling coconutty)
- sprinkle black pepper
- Celtic sea salt
- basil
- and lemon pepper to your heart's delight.
- sprinkle walnuts on top.

Midnight Asparagus Delight

To stave off the late-night munchies

- Steam eight asparagus spears
- Four mixed peppers
- ¼ jalapeño
- ½ a white onion
- Four garlic cloves
- Add a healthy chunk of ginger
- Four small vine tomatoes
- ½ tbsp. of parsley, basil and oregano
- ½ tbsp. of nutritional yeast
- 1 tbsp. of miso
- Tbsp. of coconut aminos
- $1/4^{th}$ to $1/8^{th}$ cup of Olive Oil
- Sprinkle
- Black pepper
- Celtic sea salt to season
- 1 cup of warm water
- Blend in the Vitamix until the mixture is soup-hot.

Homemade Nut and Seed Milks

Making one's own milk from Brazil nuts, Almonds, Walnuts, Macadamia nuts or Pumpkin seeds is a delightful, healing activity. It is time-consuming but worth the investment. This is the ideal midnight snack. These milks are very rich and very thick. They can be served chilled or warmed-up. If I find myself up late hanging out past mid-night, I will have a big glass jar of nut milk to keep myself full and away from the "goodies" (baddies).

- Soak 1 1/2 cups of Almonds in structured water for 4 hours. (Soak Brazil nuts and walnuts for 15 minutes, pumpkin seeds 1 hour)
- Discard original water for almonds. Use the original water for the others.
- Bring in 4-5 cups of water and blend in the Vitamix for 2 minutes.
- Strain the milk through a cheese cloth. The cheese cloth is the ultimate strainer. Give it a good proper squeeze as the cows give thanks that you are not crushing their teats. (if you have a Vita Mix then you don't need to strain any of the milks except the almond milk)
- Pour the liquid back into the Vitamix

- Bring in a spoon full of soaked and cleaned Irish moss. This is very mineral-rich but very overpowering as well, so go light to begin. If you enjoy a few more spoonfuls, go for it.

Add the following
- 1/2 tbsp. Celtic Sea Salt (this is the key ingredient to give our milks, a less boring taste but be careful with how much you initially add. As we have stated, a law of te kitchen is that you can add more but once you do, you can't subtract)
- 2 tbsp. raw honey
- 1 tbsp. coconut oil
- Few drops of vanilla extract
- 2 tbsp. of sunflower lecithin

Blend up this mix and you will have a delicious milk far better than a McDonald's vanilla shake.

Don't get frustrated if the first time it's slightly "off." You have to tweak it to your preference. As you taste it, ask yourself if adding a bit more of anything will make it a more savory experience for you. Recipes cannot always be exact because they are contingent on your taste buds. This is rather a guide for you to get in there and try your hand at it. Once you have done it 10 times then you will develop your own little tricks and know what you like.

- Do you like Quick Strawberry Milk? Add strawberries before your final blend.
- Or add a few tbsp. of Raw Cacao for Chocolate milk.
- For an even more vanilla-frappe type taste, bring in vanilla-flavored hemp protein.
- Or try adding goji berries for a Goji Love Milkshake.

Life Foods Pâté

Saving-Two-Livers at a Time Foie Gras

After we milk our ~~cows~~ nuts and seeds, are we
done? No! We still have the leftover almond or
pumpkin seed meat. Don't discard it into the
compost heap. For years, I searched for what I
could use the almond meat for. I experimented with
little imitation cake batters but I was never
convinced. But with some experimentation I got
something quite nice actually. It's almost a Foie
Gras Pate minus the livers of any living beings.

- Take the almond meat (or Brazil nut meat
  etc.) from the cheese cloth and discard half
  of it into a big bowl. You can add a little
  more later or try a different mix with the rest
  of it.
- Food process some sun flower or pumpkin
  seeds or really any combo of nuts and seeds
  and bring into the bowl [I can give you exact
  measurements but sometimes it's better to
  start low and just bring them in so you can
  get the right combo for you.]
- Begin with 1/2 cup of Brazil nuts and 1/2
  cup pumpkin seeds and 1/2 cup sunflower
  seeds.
- Add 1/2 tbsp. of Basil, Bragg's Amino
  Acids, Oregano, Mustard and Turmeric.

- Add 4 tbsp. of Apple Cider Vinegar.
- 3 tbsp. nutritional yeast.
- Two pinches of Celtic Sea Salt
- Mix it all up in a large bowl.
- Spread it thin into the bowl. The more days it sits atop the refrigerator the more it will ferment with the Apple Cider Vinegar.

Give us this day, our Daily Bread

We can make our own bread as a substitute for the harmful, starchy bread that is one of the staples of the American die-t. Through experimentation and much trial and error, I discovered this recipe.

- Place the almond meat, left over from making 4 cups of almond milk, in a big bowl. The almond meat will form the base of our bread. The almond meat by itself has no flavor but this will soon change.
- Next, for 10 minutes, we steam 5-6 broccoli florets, 10 pieces of garlic, a small white or purple onion, a red or orange pepper and a handful of mushrooms.
- Place the steamed veggies into a food processor or the vita mix.
- Add 1 tbsp. of Apple Cider Vinegar, 3 tbsps. of Braggs Amino Acids, 3 tbsps. of Balsamic Vinaigrette, 2 tbsps. of warm water, a fistful of fresh basil, 1 tbsp. of Celtic sea salt, oregano and Italian seasoning. (feel free to add other seasoning to spice it up)
- Blend all of this up for sixty seconds and voila you have your batter to flavor your almond flour.
- Pour the contents into the big bowl of almond meat. Massage the seasoning into

the almond meat until there is one consistency.

- Lay the contents — the batter — over the dehydrator trays as if it were dough.
- Dehydrate at 117 degrees for 14-16 hours.
- Dehydrate the edges for another two hours for crispy bread crust.
- Dipping this "bread" into balsamic vinaigrette, olive oil and Celtic sea salt makes for a superb snack. Or we can eat our daily bread with a pine nut-based cheese.

It's ok to be Cuckoo for Cocoa Puffs

Food Process the following
- 1 handful almonds
- 1 handful pumpkin seeds
- 1 handful walnuts or pecans or Brazil nuts
- 1 heaping tbsp. raw honey
- 1 heaping tbsp. raw cacao
- 1 heaping tbsp. sunflower lecithin
- 1 tbsp. coconut oil or butter
- Few drops vanilla

Serve as a cereal with homemade Brazil nut milk or Almond milk.

See how that comes out then experiment with your own Fruity Pebbles or Lucky Charms.

Non-Chickpea Falafels

- With the other left-over nut or seed meat, we can experiment. Food process some nuts and seeds again. Combine them with the almond meat in the master bowl.
- Tinker with this recipe some and food process 2 or 3 pieces of garlic and ¼ of an onion. Pinch of raw honey and 3 or 4 dun dried tomato. Pour in some olive oil.
- Add ½ tbsp. mustard seed, and a few other spices. Be experimental.
- Really cut back on the apple cider vinegar and nutritional yeast which give us a cheesier feel. Just add a pinch of that.
- Mix all the ingredients and then roll your mix into cute little balls, dehydrate overnight and have a nice non-legume **Falafel**. If we tweak this some, can we get something that resembles a chicken mc-nugget, Indian pakoras or vadas or maybe even an old-fashioned meatball? I leave the nomenclature intentionally vague because I don't want to suggest what the flavor is for you.
- Before naming things, I like to let people's taste buds come up with the names. What for me was a Wild Unturkey Stuffing, for

you might be a Sizzlin' Sirloin Cranberry Steak.[37]

---

[37] This is always good consolation if something does not quite turn out how you expected the first time. You can always retreat into remembering that no matter the taste, this is doing amazing things for your body.

<u>July 26th Cuban Quinoa</u>[38]

- 1 cup quinoa to 2 cups water
- Heat but do not boil.[39]
- Add 1 or 2 tbsp. of cilantro, parsley, oregano, basil, turmeric, Italian season
- Add or subtract as you see fit.
- Dice up some onions, garlic, peppers, broccoli, mushrooms, spinach, and/or sun dried tomatoes. Throw them in the pot.
- Let the quinoa take on the flavor of the ingredients by slowly cooking it for 20 minutes or so.
- At the end add some Celtic sea salt, olive oil or coconut oil to flavor.

---

[38] I got the recipe from something similar to Cuban congri aka mixed rice and beans.

[39] Sprouted quinoa is preferred and is true Life Foods but it does not take on the same flavors as cooked quinoa. By slowly cooking this ancient, protein-rich seed we are technically altering its chemical structure and life force but still receiving many of its benefits.

Coconut Quinoa

- 1 cup quinoa to 2 cups coconut milk
- Dice up onions and add.
- At the end add some Celtic sea salt, olive oil or coconut oil.
- Throw in some raisins or cranberries.
- You can try some tbsp. of cinnamon, nutmeg or anise.

Let-the-Turkeys-Run Free Wild Stuffing

- ½ cup soaked almonds
- ½ cup soaked walnuts
- ½ cup pumpkin seeds
- ½ cup chopped celery
- ½ red onion
- ½ chopped white onion
- ½-1 cup dry cranberries
- ¾ seeded raisins
- ¼ olive oil
- A few black olives depending on how much you like olives
- ¼ cup pine nuts
- 1 tablespoon rosemary
- 1 tablespoon basil
- 1 tablespoon thyme
- ½ tablespoon Celtic sea salt

- Food process all of the nuts, berries, celery and onion
- Mix all the liquid ingredients with the herbs and spices.
- Add everything into the bowl and add a little bit of water.
- Lay the servings of stuffing out into a dehydrator at 117 degrees for 16 hours then flip them and dehydrate for another 4 hours. If you are using an

oven, try at a very low temperature and check it every 20 minutes to see until it takes on the texture of Thanksgiving stuffing.

Carlo Tresca Anti-Fascist Spaghetti

- Blend ginger with warm water. Soak Kelp Noodles in this water for several hours.
- Strain the kelp noodles.
- Mix with grated or shaved down Zucchini, Yellow Squash and Cucumber (The strips mimic spaghetti.) Steam some onions and sweet peppers (optional jalapeños) and throw them all in.
- Slice up some tomatoes.
- Add olive oil, salt and freshly minced garlic to the kelp noodles.
- Stir in desired quantity and allow the kelp noodles to soak in the oil, garlic and Celtic sea salt for 10-15 minutes.
- If you desire cheesy pasta, add nutritional yeast and stir it in.
- Add black pepper and additional nutritional yeast as needed.
- Garnish with spices such as parsley.
- Add apple cider vinegar to the finished meal for a zing.
- To switch it up, you can try this recipe with the Asian ginger plum sauce for an imitation pad Thai
- Or enjoy with a more traditional Vito Russo Tomato Sauce.

Vito Russo Out of the Closet & into the Streets Tomato Sauce

- 4 vine tomatoes
- ¼ Cup olive oil
- 1 ½ tbsp. Italian seasoning
- 1 tbsp. oregano
- 1 handful fresh basil
- 2 tbsp. honey
- 1 tbsp. Apple Cider Vinegar
- 1 tbsp. Anise seed
- 1 tbsp. sun dried sea salt
- 1 ½ Cups Sun Dried Tomatoes

Blend all ingredients then add the Sun-Dried Tomatoes and Blend again.

Midnight Hot Turmeric Brazil Nut Shake

- ¼ cup of Brazil Nuts
- ¼ Cup Almonds
- 1 cup of coconut water
- ½ cup of filtered water
- Few Medjool dates
- 2 teaspoons of Mesquite powder
- 1/2 teaspoon of turmeric powder
- 1/2 teaspoon of cinnamon powder
- 1/2 teaspoon of ginger powder and/or fresh ginger
- 1/2 teaspoon of vanilla powder
- A pinch of nutmeg
- A pinch of clove
- You can add any nut or seed milk.
- Experiment with goji berry powder, maca or lucuma powder.
- Blend all this up in the vita mix and heat a bit for a wonderfully soothing hot cocoa type drink. Excellent to take the chill off.

This recipe is for the Late Night Sweet Tooth. We can partake in Life Foods at any hour. Life Foods is going to do wonderful things for us even as we sleep. The other advantage is that you really can't eat too much. Your own system will tell you when you have had enough nutrients.

130

Anti-Hospital Bed Life Protein Bars

- Food process a nut mix. Mix and match Almonds, Brazil nuts, Macadamia nuts, Pecans, Walnuts, and Pine nuts or any combination. Pumpkin seeds can be used as well. Try ½ cup of 2 or 3 of them to begin. Then you can adjust your base.
- Add goji berries, raisins, cranberries or whatever mix of those. Try ¼ cup of one or two of these.
- 2 tablespoons of sunflower lecithin
- 1-2 tablespoons of raw honey
- 1-2 tablespoons of coconut oil
- 1 tablespoon maca powder or lucuma
- Splash of organic vanilla extract
- 1 tablespoon of goji powder
- Dash of homemade Brazil nut or Almond milk
- 1 tablespoon hemp protein powder (vary it up with chocolate or vanilla flavored hemp protein)
- 1 tablespoon raw cacao or cacao nibs
- Experiment with your favorite mix. You really can't go wrong.
- Form into a bar and fit into tin foil. Stick in freezer for a few hours.
- Provides a candy bar like structure.

Nana's Bertolt Brecht Apple Sauce

- Wash apples thoroughly. Do not peel or core.
- Cut apples into 4 square slices
- Use poker to make sure all apples get blended in the Vitamix
- Add cinnamon to your heart's delight.
- In the old days people boiled the apples and then strained them through a scythe or colander. The Vitamix helps us forgo all of that. This apple sauce is unbelievably smooth and delicious. There is no sigh of the skin except in the color of the end product.

Section IV. Life Foods Extremism: 6 More Recipes that Push the Limits

I have left the best for last. I do not want to shock the reader but if you came this far you have already dared to challenge a lot of conventional ideas. I congratulate you on having an open mind and being proactive about your health. So, let's overthrow some more mainstream ideas, shall we?

I believe in being up front. If something is "weird" or different, let's examine that. If something does not taste good, let's recognize that. But does all food have to be for enjoyment? Can food be our medicine and can our medicine be our food? Treat what follows as your medicine and see where it takes you. Can we enjoy food, not for its immediate, fleeting high, which soon leaves us feeling comatose, but rather for the long-run surges in our energy and self-love?

The People's Champagne

Bacardi Chemotherapy to the Dome

(Sodium Bicarbonate Shots:
these are great for a pick me up midday)

- 2 Fresh squeezed lemons
- Juice two apples
- (or 1 Fresh Squeezed Valencia Orange but it has a sort of metal sand taste)
- 1/3 tablespoon Baking Soda
- ½ tbsp. of Citric Acid to round out the taste.
- As it fizzes up like a volcano, take it to the dome sonny!!!

You can remix this by adding some ice cubes and making this into a giant slush in the Vitamix. Great for relaxation before bed.

The Question of Coffee

Coffee is very acidic and takes its toll on the stomach over time. Coffee does indeed have a diarrheic effect but the problem is it washes away both the good and the bad bacteria. It serves as almost a battery acid for the gut. Coffee is extremely habit-forming and can cause vertigo and other uncomfortable conditions. A coffee drinker — deprived of their drug — will get a headache right on cue. Coffee is very habit forming. The withdrawal causes headaches and moodiness. If you *need* coffee, then you don't need coffee and are better off without it.

Coffee also affects the heart and circulation in a harmful way (Null 442). Other studies indicate that coffee can lower resistance to pain (Null 302).

Can we begin to substitute our coffee, especially in the morning, with some other pick-me-ups? The bicarb shots? A pinch of clove or a ginseng tea? Some hits of kombucha or fresh juiced ginger with green apple? Or some maté tea?

The best place for coffee is within the enemas that we can prepare for ourselves to filter out debris caught in the rectum in order to prevent cancerous cells from forming.

The Big UT

The Breakfast of Champions

Don't read this section if it is too much of a turnoff initially. I thought about leaving this part out because of how "unconventional" the mainstream considers Urine Therapy. Some friends have pleaded with me to delete this section but five years later, it is still here.

If you want to use it as an excuse to delay your own healing, that is your decision.

If you are not open-minded, stop right here. I am duty-bound to share this venerable secret because of the rejuvenating and circulating effect I have seen it have. I have seen it work magic in heightening people's awareness of the life around them. At other moments, I was not as impressed with the results. The point is that you must see for yourself.

According to the ancient Ayurvedic texts, urine is a natural laxative that detoxifies poisons in the system and helps absorption in the large intestine.[40] Ingesting the first morning's urine, fresh upon rising, has a powerful effect. After allowing the first few seconds of urine to be discarded, catch the rest midstream with a glass jar. This should be done in a very private way. At first this will seem

---

[40] See Dr. Vasant Lad's *Ayurveda: The Science of Self-Healing*. Twin Lakes: WI.: Lotus Press. 2009.

intimidating, but soon enough it will become a non-event. Trust this time-honored tradition employed by healers in different cultures. Give it a week or so and I dare you to tell me you are not seeing results in terms of self-awareness and heightened circulation.

The effects are also contingent upon what you are originally feeding your cells, meaning that urine therapy is not the same for a carnivore as it is for someone who is following a healthy lifestyle. Yogis and hikers have survived for days off nothing but their own urine.[41]

Urine is not excretion. Think of UT not as waste, but as a kidney-purified tea. We lose a lot of minerals in our urine. Urine therapy gives the system a second-go at absorbing essential minerals such as albumin. Albumin is essential for carrying nutrients from ingested food to the cell and waste away from the cell. Urea is an organic compound that is amazing for digestion, building the immune system and for preventing and fighting cancer. UT will help reach deeper outer space regions of the digestive system, that ordinary medicine or cleansing cannot touch.

---

[41] It is not suggested to drink someone else's urine because they have different hormones.

Urine is sterile upon exiting the body but will build up bacteria if left out over time, hence the overwhelming bad smell of urine in the street.

Urine has also been used in ancient cultures for teeth whitening and to reverse acne. While showering it can be beneficial to snort urine up both nostrils to clear the sinuses. A wasabi dish can be helpful for this task. Snorting a bit of Celtic sea salt can also be used for a runny nose through pulsating yogi breathing, but one must also be very careful with this technique.

Natural Mint Toothpaste

Mix five spoonfuls of coconut oil and five spoonfuls of baking soda. Add some drops of peppermint oil for a fresh smell or tea tree oil for even more of an antibacterial effect. Mix the toothpaste well and store in a tight jar. It stays solid in a cool room in cold weather and will be liquefied during warmer weather. This mix will help whiten your teeth.

Another Look at Dairy

The dairy industry invests hundreds of millions of dollars to convince us that we need a cow's milk for calcium despite research that proves cow milk is not a solid source of calcium.[42] Are human systems compatible with the milk produced by another species? Every notion in our minds is a reflection of our socialization and conditioning. If it's all we've ever known, it's all we can imagine.

I have heard healers who have pondered culturing cheeses and creating emulsifications with a mom's breast milk. Could this be down in a respectful way? What nutrients would we be able to access? The fact that every major media outlet seeks to scare us away from the consumption of a mother's breast milk is telling. What they cannot completely control, they seek to vilify. Why do they ignore the multitude of hormones and chemicals injected into mass-produced cow milk? This unto itself makes the nutritional value of a mother's breast milk worthy of more investigation.

---

[42] See Gary Null's blog entry "Effects of Dairy" for a well-researched forum on this topic.

Life Water

*Konstipation's Kryptonite soaked in
King Kong's Bathwater*

- 8 ounces of water
- 1 tbsp. castor oil
- 1 tbsp. MSM (METHYLSULFONYLMETHANE)
- 6-8 drops stabilized oxygen
- 1 tsp Epsom salt
- 1 tsp sodium bicarbonate (aluminum-free baking soda)
- 1 tbsp. Apple Cider Vinegar (the more you add of the ACV the more you can mask the horrific flavor.)

This is radical, often considered the most revolting of all beverages! But it does the trick!

Life Water tastes horrible but it is constipation kryptonite. It is designed to scrape and scrub the cells clean and dislodge the mold, fungus and yeast that gets jammed up in our arteries over time.

Besides Life Colloid[43] and 8-10 ounces of straight olive oil, Life Water is the most extreme concoction I have experimented with. The name sounds innocuous enough, as if it were a cousin of Vitamin

---

[43] Life Colloid is the richest of soils from the Pacific Northwest, jam packed full of healing properties.

Water. That is why I put the parenthesis with Life Water's nickname.

Life Water should be used carefully. I have overdone it and dehydrated my body in preparation for fights when I had to shed weight. I have had company and gone into the laboratory to prepare some servings of Life Water. I remember it was the NBA finals and the game was first beginning. Our poor guest was still trying to force down 8 ounces of a Life Water potion as halftime ended some 60 minutes later. Don't force it. It is not necessary. If your body is giving you that much opposition, let go.

During liver and gall bladder flushes my body has completely rejected 8-10 ounce helpings of Olive Oil. Meanwhile Louie the Plumber, Red Owl or The Bile Builder have chugged it back like it was as tasty as cold beer. Our bodies are all so unique. Never force it. We must be allowing.

One way to use Life Water is to drink it after a rough night out when you just couldn't resist some of the temptations thrown your way. Wake up to Life Water and a run, bike or swim. This routine has prompted me to evacuate up to seven times in the course of the hours that followed. Start slow with eight ounces and feel it out. You've been forewarned. You don't want to get caught out there with no mountain money (toilet paper) in the trails or in the neighborhood.

Section V. A Day in the Life

- 6 a.m. I wake up early from atop the floor I sleep!
- I jump out of bed with energy, ready to hit the pavement or grass if the weather is right. If it's cold out, I'm taking a shot of juiced ginger, lemons, cucumber and apples before the run. Maybe I'll toss some cayenne pepper in my socks to keep the happy feet moving. A shot of Apple Cider Vinegar or a bit of kombucha is invigorating. I'll take some supplements, such as MSM, magnesium, echinacea, Vitamin C or flush niacin. Just space these things out so you do not overwhelm the tummy.
- If it's an extreme day I might have 10 ounces of Life Water.
- Oil Swishing and Pulling for first 10-20 minutes of my run.
- I aim for 5 to 8 miles barefoot. I end with yoga and handstands.
- 8 a.m. I'm back at the Life Foods Headquarters. I wrap my gall bladder and liver up in some Castor Oil packs and apply some heat to do some Outer Galactic Cleansing.
- I prepare a fresh juice or a ginger, lemon, honey tea.

- I make a potent, filling smoothie.
- 9 am I'm off to work with my granny bag.
- All morning, I sip from my glass jars.
- 2 p.m. I dig into the heartier blended soups
- Before hitting the 1 4 9 boxing club, I take some hits of People's Champagne.
- 5 pm I'm in the ring dancing, moving and slipping.
- 7 pm I'm showering up.
- If there is time in the day, I'll do a yoga class to complete the trifecta.
- For a night cap, I have more blended soup.
- I have a People's Hummus or a Mango Salsa ready to go and I dip a cucumber or a nori sheet in there.
- I end the night with peppermint tea, another Castor Oil Pack and a lilac essential oil, Hydrogen Peroxide Foot Soak.
- Reading, studying. Mediation.
- I am in bed between 11 pm and 1 am.
- I repeat this routine the next day while remaining conscious of over-training and learning to listen to my body.

Section VI. Debunking Myths

Capitalism is a myth-making machine. The number of half-truths and clichés that pass as science is remarkable. As a result of my transformation, I've been called crazy, an extremist, anorexic, gaunt, frail, a weirdo, a hippie and the like. Especially for those of us coming from working class and oppressed communities, we are going against family and cultural traditions. In Section IV. I will take on eight of the most common lies that you will come across, in order to intellectually arm you for the adventure you have embarked upon.

Myth #1

"You will have no protein if you give up meat."

When I go to purchase a thirteen or eighteen punch combination salad, the cashier inevitably asks, "with or without protein?"

Why do we equate meat with protein? Why do we equate protein with athletic prowess? It is the healthy organic carbohydrates that are delivering the building blocks we need for strength and endurance. An overemphasis on proteins may make you "buff" but can also render you quite bulky and overburden your system. Remember we are *Shedding that which is not Us*, not hiding toxins beneath layers of muscles. We want to de-bulk, not over-bulk. Many star athletes in the boxing, football and wrestling world appear invincible because of their muscle volume but inside their pancreas and colons are crying out in anguish for relief. I knew a wrestler at the top of his game who suddenly discovered a tumor that was so large it was protruding from his stomach into the nerves in his back. He died within two months of discovering the growth.

There are plenty of plant-based sources of protein, such as collard greens, broccoli, spinach, bok choy, okra, amaranth, hemp, quinoa, nuts, and sprouted seeds. Hemp protein is great with smoothies. When we are plant-strong, we are in control of our futures!

The people who love you will repeat the following ad nauseam: "What? No meat? You are going to wither away. You'll have no protein." Many of my top detractors suffer from diabetes, obesity and ulcers, yet they worry about me? Recognize that this most often comes from a place of love, a desire to protect and a fear of change. Stay the path.

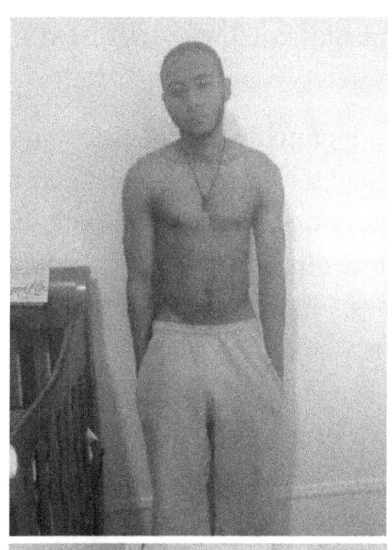

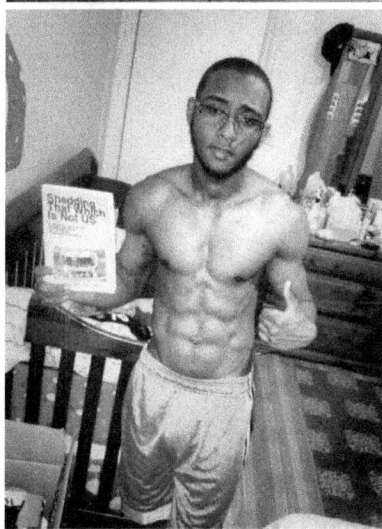

Nicolás transformed his mindset and body in two months' time

The artist, Nicolás Fernandez, known in the hip hop world as Jayzoon, changed his life style and saw breath-taking results in eight weeks. Does he look like he lacks protein?

There are false hierarchies about lean proteins that we should not buy into, such as the supposition that red meat is the worst meat, with pork being the forerunner. According to this misinformation, the "leaner" fleshes, like chicken and turkey then follow, with fish being the healthiest. Who made this up? This is anti-scientific. Flesh is flesh. We should stay clear of anything that has a heartbeat or a face, for both ethical and trophic reasons. All flesh is putrid, decays within the body and can take months to pass through. This is what triggers the *Itis*.[44] Never again do we want to feel this unpleasant, cumbrous feeling.

Does cow flesh or chicken flesh have protein? Yes. However, the protein utilization is very low because the body cannot break down the flesh. And "animal sources of protein often contain large amounts of synthetic hormones, saturated fats, antibiotics, pesticide residues, nitrates, toxic waste, mercury and a host of other potentially harmful ingredients."[45]

Blended soups and smoothies are amazing. It's like pouring the mineralization and protein into your

---

[44] Slang term for the feeling after you have ingested a big meal and need to sleep off the effects.
[45] Gary Null. Get Healthy Now. NY: Seven Stories Press. 2006.

veins. Within fifteen minutes, the nutrients are distributed and absorbed throughout your body. Meanwhile, a slab of filet mignon will take six to eight hours to pass through your system. In fact, much of it will never be absorbed but will become putrid in the body. Think of babies' digestive systems. Why do they take in purees? After the teeth, there is nothing to protect the gut. A good measure of whether or not something is Life Foods is asking yourself an hour after eating, are you ready to move? If the answer is no, you have probably overloaded your digestive system. Over time, indigestion is very dangerous.

Myth #2

"Our metabolism slows down as we get older."

According to this outdated mode of thinking, the die is cast. Why would anyone put up a fight if they are already damned?

How you treat your body dictates the rate at which you can digest and absorb nutrients. We are not condemned to become old and washed up. We are self-determining.

Investigative journalist Grace Halsell reached similar conclusions in *Los Viejos: Secrets of Long*

Life from the Sacred Valley.[46] Halsell went to live with the indigenous people of Vilcabamba, Ecuador in the Andean mountains. Their lifestyle, rustic and simple, was protected from all of the stresses and contamination that came with "modernity." They had no access to television, ice-cream, the market economy and sugars. They were living consistently living to be older than 100 years of age. The people of Vilcabamba had one of the highest rates of centenarians on the planet. Inner-peace, pure foods, an active love of life and a relationship with nature were the keys to their longevity. It sounds so simple. But, how complicated simple living becomes in a world mis-guided and warped by the wills of small, egotistical, haughty pigs who have deprived us of nature!

A demented prison experiment in Jim Crow Mississippi in 1915 demonstrated how quickly death by starchicide could afflict people. A New York City-based bacteriologist, Joe Goldburg, sought to understand a skin disease known as pellagra. Following leads on studies he had conducted in "insane asylums," Goldburg enrolled eleven male prisoners into a study on a plantation farm. He promised them freedom if, for six months, they ate only "white bread, corn pone, hominy grits, sweet potatoes, salt pork, cane syrup, cabbage and

---

[46] Emmaus, PA: Rodale Press, Inc. 1976.

coffee" (Dufty 128). Predictably, within weeks, the prisoners developed back pain, headaches, stomach aches, dizziness and red lesions under their scrotum. Pellegra was indeed a skin condition caused by diet.

Goldburg's experiment was a Southern, white supremacist version of Morgan Spurlock's 2004 documentary *Supersize Me.* Hoping to show the harmful effects of fast food, the film director ate McDonalds for thirty days straight. By the second week, Spurlock was bloated and incapable of even achieving an erection with his girlfriend. These experiments prove that metabolism or oxygen consumption is affected by what we put into our bodies.

And the inverse is true. Those that let go of starches, dairy and meat can oxygenate and hydrate the cells and undo years and decades of damage. Those that have begun the Life Journey know that there is a whole new you within, waiting to be birthed. A few weeks and months have changed many peoples' lives. Sustaining this lifestyle is a lifelong challenge.

Myth #3

"Health problems run in my family. Disease is hereditary."

Again, this is so fatalistic, no? In the overwhelming majority of cases, this is an absolutely false supposition. Fertility, a smooth menstrual cycle and hormone regulation are all greatly impacted by stress, poor eating habits, mineral deficiencies, a lack of exercise, contamination in the water supply, alcohol, cigarettes and other environmental factors.[47] The truth is that poor eating and living habits run in the household resulting in common instances of male or female reproductive issues. Almost every working-class American family experiences instances of heart disease, colon cancer, acid reflux, gastritis, high blood pressure, high cholesterol, diabetes, chronic pain and blood clots. We are all united by the over-occurrence of these illnesses.

When I go to family reunions it's predictable. We gather around seemingly endless family recipes and a half hour later everyone is complaining about belly aches and searching for a couch to sleep off the fatigue. I was once part of this routine. My recovery came in the form of training to work it off. But I was running on a treadmill. I didn't want to keep feeling heavy and lethargic. Director Aiyana Elliott's brilliant documentary "Simply Raw" documents how some average Americans — who are up against all odds — are able to reverse their

---

[47] Null. 2006. Page 759.

diabetes in a relatively short amount of time.[48] I think it's important to witness one another's transformation to believe that we too can wrest back control over our lives.

I won't sit by and watch the beloved die off. In the words of Big Bill Haywood "I haven't read Marx's *Capital*, but I have the marks of capital all over my body." In other words, our communities might not immediately recognize the source of their suffering but they carry the scars. Our role as organizers is to elucidate the unnatural origins of the pain because this is not living! We deserve and must demand better!

Myth #4

"Cancer and other dis-eases are uncontrollable, permanent and non-reversible."

Don't believe the hype about cancer being a death sentence. The greatest way to control people is through fear. The Dis-ease Establishment defeats people before they even dare to heal themselves.

The average American consumes 140 pounds of sugar per year.[49] Sugar "drains and leeches the body of precious vitamins and minerals through the

[48] Aiyana Elliot's documentary released in 2009.
[49] *The Truth about Cancer*. Part IV.

demand its digestion, detoxification and elimination make upon one's entire system."[50] Starches and sugars feed cancer. Life Foods purifies our inner terrain depriving cancerous cells of the toxicity that they feed off. Life Foods goes to war against neoplasm, the out of control, abnormal tissue or tumors that have become cancerous.[51]

For some potential self-healers, the withdrawal will be too challenging initially. For others, the conditioning is too thorough. Some Americans will have to reach rock bottom — developing kidney stones, for example, vertigo or an enlarged prostate — before they realize how serious dis-ease is.

This can be very frustrating for the person trying to help the affected individual heal. The watchwords are Patience and Perseverance.

We can get away with murder on the body in our 20's but by our 30's these conditions start to catch up with us and by our 40's and 50's they pounce on us. I adapted Marcus Garvey's formulation about organizing in Harlem at the beginning of the 20th century to the task before us:

If all else fails with a hardheaded family member or friend

---

[50] William Dufty. p. 137)

[51] For a full discussion of stopping cancer in its tracks see page 101 of Dr. David and Annie Jubb's *Secrets of an Alkaline Body*. Berkeley: North Atlantic Books. 2004.

Their own misery
may prove to be the supreme organizer.

At 41, Louie "the Plumber" was adamant that "the berry-picking thing," as he facetiously and derisively called it, was not for him. After suffering from high blood pressure and then a "sudden" heart attack, his mind opened up. Near death experiences have a way of encouraging reflection.

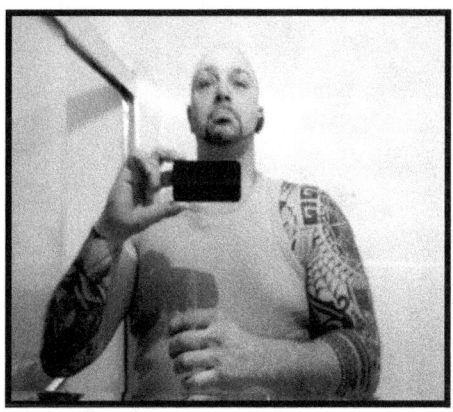

A heart attack waiting to happen

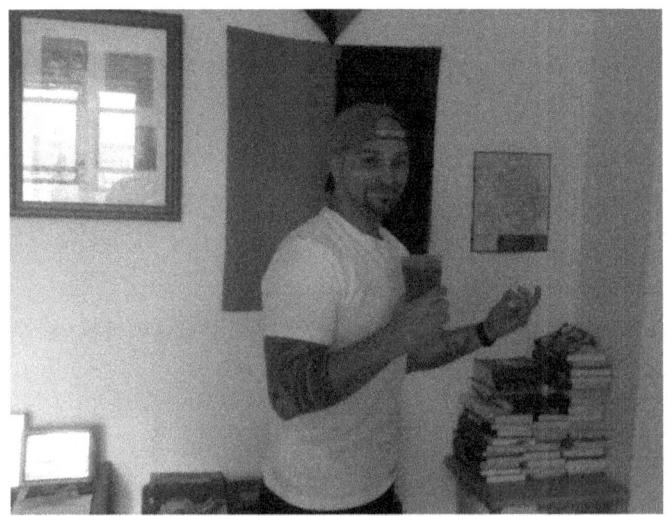

6 Months and 85 Pounds later

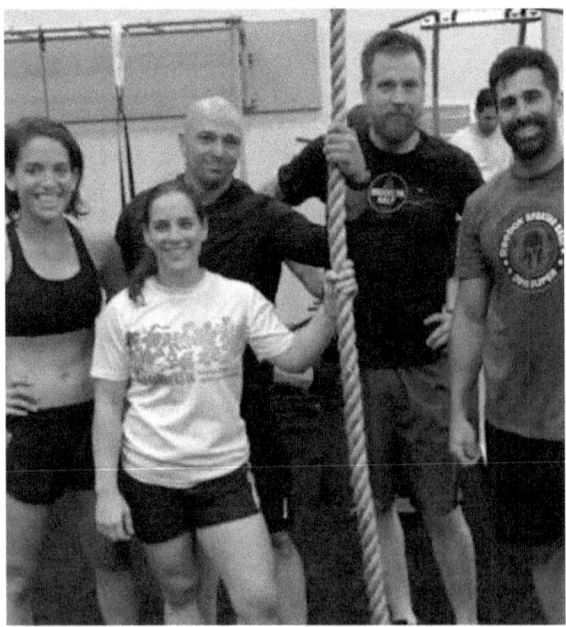

The Selfie-King with his Spartan Team

As a veteran of Desert Storm, "the Plumber" was no stranger to discipline and routine. He embraced Life Foods almost 100%, which is undeniably challenging for a new comer. The results were astounding. In 6 months, he shed 85 lbs. After running hundreds of miles on the open road, the Plumber was reborn. At 44, he is the youngest he has ever been. Today Louie, or the Selfie-King, competes in Spartan races across the country.

If your time is not now, maybe you'll find an opening in the years to come. There is no judgment. Is there a rush? Is there urgency? It is plain to see that there is a collective crisis but it has to come from you. There are no liberators. The motivation has to come from deep within. Don't wait until rock bottom to challenge yourself.

Myth #5
"I Can't Afford This"

This is not entirely a myth. There is immense truth in this statement. Tupac Shakur and Michael Jackson were all too accurate when they both sang "They don't really care about us." There are no Whole Foods or Trader Joes in isolated, oppressed neighborhoods. Furthermore, the prices at these stores downtown are exorbitant.

We live in Food Deserts. For the most part, the foods introduced in this book are not part of our modern identity. Indeed, you will be a trail blazer and trend setter. Prepare for a barrage of criticism and enormous challenges.

Yes, there will be new expenses incurred. Bee pollen at $12.99 a bottle and flax seed oil at $19.99 for a small bottle is not cheap. What are some strategies we can explore to overcome this? Let's maintain a sense of revolutionary optimism. Think of this transformation as a reorganization of priorities. Instead of going out to eat three times a week or going to a bar a few times on the weekend, can we cut these outings down to one? Balance is essential.

The price excuse can be a cop out for some individuals. Let's be direct. Who wants to give up all of the mouth-watering, "good stuff?" What's your motivation? You have to be self-driven to do this. Too many times, I've heard friends retort: "What do I care? I have to die at some point." But when the gout, inflammation or kidney stones hit, I don't see them laughing at the kombucha anymore. How many hard-headed, flippant, devil-may-care type characters are literally starving for change? Can they begin to let go? *Fat, Sick and Nearly Dead* is a great place to start for the everyday blue-collar worker. Joe Cross' 2010 documentary follows his journey and that of an obese truck driver as they begin juicing and saying no to harmful foods.

When I conduct workshops and engage in one-on-one conversations, the self-defense mechanisms flare up. I am shocked by how many people I come across who have "nut allergies." Why are nut allergies so common? An allergy is the overwhelming of the cell with certain elements the cell cannot handle. Why don't people have hamburger or hot dog allergies? Or is that what a tummy ache is? Could the nut sensitivity have to do with the chemical alteration of the cellular structure due to vaccines? Are the nuts picking up microtoxins and aflatoxins when they are cultivated packed and transported? Or are some Americans semi-consciously justifying they're not budging one inch from their Standard American Diet? Very S.A.D. indeed. There is so much fear of change. All of the scientific evidence is not in but I suspect the answer lies somewhere within these three explanations. It just does not add up that so many people have a negative response to something that grows wild in nature while they can simultaneously ingest its diametrical opposite. Dependency manifests itself in many different ways.

The point is not to wage an internal insurrection overnight. Begin simple. Integrate some dried mangoes or Brazil nuts. Sip on Strawberry

Electrolyte Lemonade all morning. UPS cannot air-drone deliver you your salvation.

Gardening is obviously just fantastic but for so many of us city dwellers it's not an option. Go to Farmer's Markets, buy organic the best you can, and start growing what you can.

Myth #6

"I don't have time."

Beware of excuses. Paradigm-shifting is unsettling. Individuals starving for mineralization unconsciously and semi-consciously erect self-defense mechanism, spurting out: "You don't know how much I work" or "I'm already overwhelmed." Life Foods will not overwhelm you. They will free you. It's the greatest investment you can make.

The same individuals who say they don't have time for a jog are out "running" the streets until five in the morning with their crew, showing what their true priorities are.

Less Hangin'
More Training.

Earn the right to hang out. The nine to five monotony and drudgery already explains away every form of escapism but we have to bear down. How good does it feel when you arrive at a house party or a social gathering and you can feel that soreness and hard work that you put into your work out? That's how I ride. Let's not just admire World Cup soccer players and marvel at boxer's bodies on TV. Forge that body for yourself. Too many people give up too early.

You've got to earn that rest
or it doesn't feel right.

Create a life style amenable to your vision. I am an educator and mentor positioned within the largest public university system of the U.S. to open up minds and arteries. I do not work a 9 to 5 job. This is quite intentional. The workaholic lifestyle so many of us are forced into swallows our vitality. To paraphrase the German poet, Bertolt Brecht, "our very survival is a miracle."

Worse yet, if you are in the Non-Profit Industrial Complex or union organizing world, you are often required to work a 60+ hour week. I have worked with some school principals and borne witness to the weight they have gained after their first year of taking on this overwhelming, inhuman job. I am also a full-time father to a beautiful thirteen-year-old. There are always challenges to be navigated. Making excuses are the surest guarantee you will never reach your goal.

Life Foods prep is time consuming. This is not for the scrawny-hearted. You are obligated to get in the kitchen and get your hands dirty. But the energy you invest here will replicate itself in every other facet of your life. It's an investment in your future that will reverberate into the decades that await you.

Because of my schedule, I do daily Life Foods prep.

Once I reached this high
Why would I want to come down off it?
I fell in love with the feeling,
the boundless energy and the mental alertness.

But let's say you are imprisoned by a 9 to 5 job or worse yet a 9 a.m. to 9 p.m. job. Take advantage of your weekends to sprout buckwheat, sunflower seeds, and quinoa. Make a gallon of Electrolyte Lemonade. Pack the dehydrator with kale chips and quinergy bread. Juice for a few days. Prepare some monster smoothies every other night for the morning.

It is also of critical importance that you surround yourself with like-minded people. The mantra and starting point of Alcoholics Anonymous is "We are addicts." Food has had a grip on our lives. If you are aiming to dive over freshly-discovered horizons, take time for yourself and surround yourself with positive-minded people who can keep you honest and balanced. If in the recent past you had a habit of going to Happy Hour after work with a group of colleagues, your new goals might mark a break in that pattern. Plan accordingly. Make alternative plans. Invite your old crew along for the ride, to yoga, to Turkish and Russian bathhouses, to acupuncture, to make smoothies together or to try a cycling class. Decipher for yourself who is going to infinitely compliment you and who is going to infinitely complicate your mission. A million people will swear up and down they are ready to make the ultimate sacrifices and implement deep-seated changes but only those who are integral will stay the path. Prepare yourself for victory and weed out the negative influences. This may appear overly harsh, but your own healing will ultimately inspire them to make profound changes in their own lives. We cannot position ourselves to heal others, until we have healed ourselves.

We will need all the help we can get confronting the temptations that haunt us wherever we go in this society. There are times I am out for a run and a whiff of Cuban *congri* (rice and beans) just stops me in my tracks and transports me back to Havana. A sniff of pizza or some French fries and hamburgers drenched in ketchup makes me daydream. Wade in the enticement.

Dominate the temptations
so that they do not dominate you.

Cravings are psychological though they do have a physiological component as well. Chemically laden fast-foods are quick fixes but what do they do for you in the long term? Recognize them for what they are — drugs.

Myth #7

"You are going against the doctor's orders. This is not well-balanced."

One twenty-four-year-old young woman struggling with Crohn's pleaded with me: "Danny I don't want to say goodbye to a normal, balanced way of life! I want to keep living." I thought this was an interesting choice of words. She was having 6 to 8 nearly uncontrollable, diarrheic episodes a day! This was not living! Our starting point should be that no one has to lead an existence that entails so much suffering.

Is sacrificing some immediate gratification for a lifetime of liberation worth it? That is a question only you can address for yourself. Trust me, what today appears like absolute self-deprivation, within time, becomes a rhythm you will never want to give up.

Life Foods is the perfect balance because it allows for proper cellular respiration. Starches, meats, dairies and fired foods produce fungus, mold and yeast in the body. From the womb through kindergarten, through freshman year away at college, we have learned to stuff our tummies with heavy starches such as bread, pasta, oats and rice. Can you stay clear of all grains? They dress up breads in such fancy packages to convince us that they are healthy. Go beyond the lying labels and read the ingredients. They have high fructose corn syrup and chemical additives and cause blockages.

I have done workshops where people are excited to learn how to halt diabetes and reverse heart conditions. They show up so adamant. They say: "Yes yes we will do anything to heal." But when I introduce the idea of saying No to harmful things, they shut down. "But wait. I am Dominican. Rice, beans and chicken is my national flag. I can't do this." So, are you giving up before you have tried?

I'm called an extremist all the time.
I say that the state of health of our people
is what is extreme.
I am only as radical as reality.

Doctors receive little to no genuine nutritional training. According to Dr. Colin Campbell less than 5% of doctors had exposure to holistic methods of healing. Most "experts" scoff at the ideas that are put forward in this book. By trusting them, we hand over control of our destiny to them at our own peril. Do you trust "your" politicians? Do you trust your teachers? Why then would you trust the yes-men of the medical industry? They are not healers. They are pill-pushers. They are bribed butchers. They are organ-thieves. Whether they are naïve or conniving cutters, they are cutters nonetheless. This is not a moral judgment of their persona but rather a sober look at their biased training. Trust them if you have been in an accident and have a broken limb. They can reset broken bones. But for internal healing, who do I trust? Me! That's who!

Myth #8
"There are no diesel vegans."[52]

I have heard this comment more than once travelling across this country. I consider myself well-positioned to debunk some of these stereotypes about vegans and raw foodists. The typical class portrait of a vegan in this society is a white person of privilege from some hippie-skippie, suburban background who fails to bathe himself properly.[53] They are rarely considered to be athletes.

We are trying to bring a new flavor, aesthetic and feel to Life Force healing and make it attractive to our communities. Some of the resistance we see comes from people justifiably feeling that "this is a white people's or rich people's way of eating and what I see is them encroaching upon my

---

[52] Diesel is slang for being strong or having defined muscles.

[53] In their case they don't just need Life Foods, they need an ideological make over that more intimately acquaints them with how we are living on this side of the class divide.

neighborhood trying to force us to move out." Change has to come from the hood for the hood. It will not come from without. Major props and a Wellness Salute! to RBG Fitness, Stik Man, Revolutionary Fitness, Queen Afua, Supa Nova Slom and other health warriors who have emerged in our communities to empower people. Their example is the wave of the future.

People tell me my lifestyle is not sustainable. Is how we are living and dying now sustainable? The predictions are that this generation coming of age will be the first to die younger than their parents.[54] The Center for Disease Control and Prevention provides evidence that "American Bellies are Getting Bigger" every day. They found that the average American waistline has increased 54% in the past few years.[55] How much more suffering do we have to experience?

I want to emphasize how tempted I feel every day by death foods. I often see vegans' faces filled when revulsion when they come close to meat. I am not repulsed by hot dogs and meatloaf. I actually rather quite enjoy them. But they were doing damage to me and the planet, so I made an adjustment. I do not come from an ethical vegan background. I come

---

[54] "Hungry for Change."

[55] Parramore, Lynn Stuart. *Alternet* "American Bellies are Getting Bigger." September 24th 2014.

from nothing. I come from the bottom. I come from poverty. I was raised by a single mother who worked whatever job was necessary and hustled to pay the rent. If you listen to my mother today, you would swear I was raised on a healthy balanced diet. I already mentioned what she was able to access in order to feed "Big D," as my family has always called me. I don't fault her. She was busy trying to survive and make a dollar out of 15 cents. The healthiest meal I remember is "Chef salads" but even that was packed with cold cuts, cheeses and the base was the wimpiest most genetically modified vegetable of them all, iceberg lettuce. We were in survival mode. My favorite food from an early age was free food. I can remember being at a truck stop and if someone had left a bunch of untouched food on their plate I would take advantage.

I want to end where I began to remind the reader that anything is possible. I don't remember having any reference point on nutrition until I was already in my mid-20's. The few times I did see my old man, I have vivid images of eating chocolate covered donuts for breakfast. He was a life-time coffee drinker and cigarette smoker. My father, George Bernard Shaw died of lung cancer when I was 17. I never really had the opportunity to know him well. How I would have liked to have known him better and walked the streets with him to learn from his myriad life experiences. "A man's man," a veteran's veteran, he was well loved by his contemporaries and was even voted the mayor of his home town, Maynard, Massachusetts. But he was not elected mayor on a nutritional platform, that is for sure. He would have derided any idea of trying to live healthy.

In college, I was infamous for sneaking into the all-you-can-eat cafeteria. When I could no longer sneak in, I reckoned if I could not beat them, I would join them. I was hired as a dishwasher in the back of the cafeteria and I was entitled to a free meal plan. I lifted a lot of weights and weighed in at an imposing 250 pounds. That was eleven years ago. Who I am today, is not who I was then. Who will I be in another decade? Where will this Life Foods journey take me? Where will it take you?

Section VII. Harmonizing Your Body and Being

Shedding that which is Not Us would not be complete without addressing a truly whole-body approach to the healing that lies before us. It would be infantile to think that our die-t is the silver bullet to cure all of our problems. But believe it or not, I've heard self-described "gurus" who argued that every social or psychological issue could be solved through our nutrition. I believe our subsistence can be the basis for healing from "ADHD" or "schizophrenia" or "Irritable Bowel Syndrome" but this has to be down in tandem with emotional healing as well.[56] We have to address what's in between the ribs, but also what's in between the ears. I felt compelled to include a closing section on mental health and spiritualty because of the intense imbalances I've noticed in different nutritional circles. Denial is a powerful thing. How convenient to recite healing formulas for others, yet fail to reflect on one's own shortcomings. Listening is more integral to self-care and self-growth than talking.

Insomnia, depression, anxiety, schizophrenia and other "mental illnesses" are sure manifestations that something is out of whack. I believe that the emotional must align with the spiritual, political and nutritional. If one element is out of place, we cannot have harmony in our broader being.

In so many cases insomnia, addiction, and overeating are merely dramatic manifestations of pain lurking deep within. Pain unresolved is pain

---

[56] I put these terms in quotes because I truly believe they are inventions of the Disease-Establishment to deepen our dependency on this or that medication. Several generations ago or today in the less "Globalized" (read Americanized) regions of the Amazon or the Philippines, are societies labeling children "hyperactive" or "depressed" the way doctors do in the U.S.? A great deal of money is being made off our suffering. As this book posits, medications are an absolute last resort.

that continues to haunt us in some way, shape or form. Dr. Gabor Mate has conducted studies showing that children with trauma were 1600 times more likely to become addicts than children who were not.[57] In the case of almost all the women in my family, and many of the men, this has been the exact scenario. The war against denial — taking the pain head on — is at the center of healing, otherwise, every healthy adjustment will leave you as incomplete as ever.

I do activities in my classes at the City University of New York to draw out some of this pain in a collective, therapeutic way. Once I have established rapport and trust with the group, I facilitate an activity where everyone in the class can anonymously submit a life issue that has caused them pain and about which they want to receive support and advice. I have included one anonymous student's response that captures the essence of the healing we have to do, both within and beyond the gut. Her poem "Losing Control" drastically captures how eating is connected to trauma.[58]

"Losing Control"

I can't seem to control myself.
I look in the mirror and I don't like what I see.

---

[57] *In the Realm of Hungry Ghosts. North* Atlantic Books. 2010.
[58] She asked that her name not be used.

I don't like what I've become.
This person trapped under
mounds of skin and flesh.
Suffocated by my own fat,
body swelling beyond its proportion
and everything seems out of control.
I'm hurting myself.
With every bite I conceal the pain of a past
and secure the torture in the present.
I hurt myself.
I walk and my body aches, my knees crack and pop
with pressure of this weight.
I feel the 180 and the 220,
the 306 and the 368 weighing down on my ribs.
My breaths are becoming shallower
and I feel this pain and I hear you when you say,
"You young lady are obese
and in grave danger of diabetes"
but that means nothing to me
when I'm home alone
and my soul is aching for relief.
My mouth crying out for instant gratification
and the fridge is taunting me.
CALLING MY NAME,
SPEAKING IN TOUNGUES
and I can't seem to control
the need to wrap myself
in Häggen-Dazs and Breyers,
sweet chocolate truffles, warm brownies,

platos de arroz con gandules y pasteles,
home fries with scrambled eggs,
chicken and broccoli,
a grande caramel flavored Frappuccino
with one shot of espresso, extra ice,
a shot of caramel syrup,
topped off with whipped cream.
I'm sick you know,
Hurting myself this way,
sitting on my bed with two pints of ice cream,
craving some sort of gratification,
but bite after bite,
my vanilla bean soaked tongue
no longer feels pleased or satisfied, but sick.
I still hear the taunting,
but it's no longer coming from my fridge.
My mind is mocking me.
"You have no self-control."
It says, "Keep eating, kill yourself."
Its tone switches, almost caring,
"Why do you do this to yourself?
Don't you love yourself?"
and I want to scream the answer,
Shout It Out, but I'm tired.
There's no fiber in Pop Tarts
and I shift my weight and hope tonight
is not the night my heart gives out.
I cry and hope tonight is not the night
gluttony damns this girl.

Why do you do this to yourself?
That questions repeats itself,
this question becomes my new mantra
when I'm stuffed and about to explode.
When the tears are falling,
my mantra becomes a whisper,
caressing me until I fall asleep.
Why do you do this to yourself?
Or better yet, why do mothers wake their children
up at 3 in the morning,
disturbing little bodies,
slipping on socks
and taking them to crack houses
on East 115th street and Lexington Avenue?
Why do step-uncles create games,
where their penises meet in little girl's mouths?
Why do daddies hit?
Why do boys get bashed for liking other boys?
Why do citizens of flooded cities
become discarded?
Why do past pains become present battles,
and future victories?"

I use this student's testimony to ask other students about addictions and their origins. There is a great deal of healing that we have to do on an emotional level or little else will ever make sense.

The only way out of it
is through it.

To ascribe to Life Foods the power to correct all social ills is ridiculous. Clearing away compact fecal matter constitutes a gut-saving individual transformation. But if we stop there, we will fall well short of individual, never mind collective, liberation. What work have you done to accept, to forgive and to heal? We are as dark as our darkest secrets. Coming from a family of incest, sexual abuse survivors and addicts, I always emphasize the need to:

Unearth the pain
or it will ride you
run you and
ruin you
right to the grave.

Section VIII. The Only Genuine Revolution

The fact that there is such an intense economic, racial and nutritional segregation still in place in the Toxic States of America in 2015 is but another reminder that this system is broken. Our work in Life Foods is to bridge the nutritional divide and provide life-bearing foods to all. We don't need another organic market in Hollywood. We need an affordable market on my block, 149th and Jackson Ave.[59]

---

[59] For those wanting to read deeper into the concept of Food Deserts and the lack of access that our communities have, a

In his preteen years, my son overheard a comment about the "C-word." Too innocent to be introduced to the ugly four-letter word, I told him the ugliest word in the English language is "Conventional." At "health" food stores, the produce is divided up between conventional and organic foods? In our neighborhoods from South Central to South Chicago to Roxbury, we don't have an organic option in the supermarkets. Conventional is double-speak for food that has been chemically altered. Who would have imagined in ancient times or today in the mountains of Chefchaouen, Morocco or in the Amazon that we would feed our children vegetables and fruits laden with pesticides, herbicides, preservatives and other toxins?

In *The China Study* Dr. Colin Campbell of Cornell painstakingly researched the massive increase in cancer cases in the United States.[60] At the turn of the 20th century, roughly one in one hundred Americans suffered from cancer. Today despite all of our technological "advancements," the rate is one in ten Americans who will develop cancer (or much higher according to other studies). Dr. Campbell attributes this to the over consumption of meat

---

2010 study by Michael Correll published by the *Duke Journal of Gender Law & Policy* entitled "Getting Fat on Government Cheese: The Connection Between Social Welfare Participation Gender and Obesity in America," is one place to start.

[60] Dallas: Benbella Books. 2005.

proteins and all of the junk that is pumped into what we perceive as "food."

Is the United States the most advanced society or the most backward? Never before has any society consumed so many anti-depressants, sleep medicine and other pills. Never in human history were there so many diagnoses of ADHD, depression, PTSD and a host of other preventable conditions.

The jingoistic slogan "God Bless America" is devoid of meaning. May the creator watch over and manifest itself in all life. May we emanate out love and solidarity to all of the life that surrounds us.

The most beautiful word among us incidentally begins with a C as well, "common," as in community, our commonalities, communion, and the common (wo)man. How can any future not be based on our collective empowerment and liberation? Just as the powers that be have undertaken great efforts to deprive us of wild strawberries, they have also sought to deprive us of the only tools that will return those wild strawberries to collective control. "If you are afraid of communism" — a collective system of control over the wealth that is generated in a society — "you are afraid of yourself."[61] Just as every effort

---

[61] Quote by the 21 year-old Chairman of the Black Panther Party in Chicago, murdered by the Chicago Police Department in his sleep in 1969.

has been made to get us hooked on addictive sugars and starches, every effort has been made to wipe out any alternative to a social system based on the hoarding of wealth by a tiny group of billionaires. Can you imagine that the Walton family, the owners of Walmart, are worth $93 billion dollars?[62] This is the equivalent of what over 40% of American workers are collectively worth. Despite anti-communism being the unofficial religion of this country, the words communism and capitalism continued to be the most googled words of 2013.[63] Humanity is hungry for change. The only way forward is an economy that is centrally planned and organized by popular representation by the most oppressed sectors of society. Anything short of this is pie in the sky and Life Foodarians will continue to be a tiny minority, isolated from the multitude of people who cannot afford this lifestyle.

The question of how to popularize Raw Foods and move beyond the perception that we are some kombucha-sippin,' sun dried tomato dog-flipping fruitcakes is important. The essential question however, is the question of power and how to seize state power. It is important to set the record straight once again in this conclusion. I honestly don't care

---

[62] *Forbes 500.* "Richest Families of the Forbes 400." from 1982-1988

[63] Taken from a speech by ANSWER Coalition spokesperson Brian Becker.

what you eat, if you are down to eat up the ruling class, you are on the right side of history. I have my priorities straight.

Revolutions do not occur in individual digestive tracts, minds or refrigerators. It is great when we can take individual or better yet collective steps towards healthy living, but the ultimate goal is the building of a society that cares and provides for the nutritional advancement and empowerment of all of us. These topics are addressed in more depth in my other books, at LiberationNews.org and LiberationSchool.org.

This is the day to day work of Revolutionary Fitness, the ANSWER Coalition, Justice First, Women Organized to Resist and Defend (WORD) and the Party for Socialism and Liberation. Check it out. Organize! Let's get free!

Section IX. Conclusion: "The Truth is Always Concrete."[64]

How's the tummy looking? How's the blood flowing? Is the largest organ in the body aka the skin radiant? Is your energy bursting out and inspiring others? Are you flying out of bed in the morning? How is your reproductive health and menstrual cycles? Are you bushy-tailed, radiating

---

[64] Quote by the German dialectician Hegel.

out good energy or always wondering why you feel so lethargic? Are the evacuations effortless, light, and fluffy and bright colors? Is your smile infectious? How's the bedroom action going? How's your flexibility? This is all proof of how you are treating and training your body.

"The truth is always concrete," and if your poop is like concrete, then the truth is you are in dire need of change.

Every theory and program has to be tested in practice. I don't disparage anyone's nutritional or athletic regiment. What I have outlined in this book is what has worked for me. I love dabbling in and trying different things. Let your own internal balance and stomach guide you, not a philosophy. Don't be rigid and dogmatic. I understand that some people feel bringing in some organic, "ethically-treated" meat compliments them and their goals.[65] But experience Life Foods, before concluding what works for you. Then evaluate all of the options and make your own informed decision.

Don't miss the opportunity to reach new heights and to live on a permanent natural high. Who I am today, is not who I will be in five years. A Life Foodist, like a revolutionary, is a pioneer and never

---

[65] Not sure killing a living being could ever be considered ethical but this is a perennial debate.

stops growing. Probe, question and try everything, then draw your own independent conclusions.

Where will your travels bring you? How exciting to dive over infinite horizons! In the words of the immortal Nuyorican poet Pedro Pietri: "If you don't become a missing person every now and then, you will never know who the hell you are." Retreat into yourself. Build up that base that will empower you to deal more gently and poignantly with the challenges and human relationships you have. "Timidity never made it in history."[66] You have to be willing to experiment and explore to discover what works for you.

Thank you for reading and opening up your mind to my wild life style. Come join me anytime on 1 4 9 for some yoga, boxing, training, healing, barefootism and vitamixing. Let's build this Life Foods family! Let's forge a new world! I got your back!

---

[66] Sam Marcy. Founder of Worker's World Party.

Section X. Services and Contact Info

Danny Shaw Facebook

DRS33@Columbia.edu

- Seminars & Group Kitchen Cleaning & Training
- Weight Loss Programs
- Yoga, meditation, and anti-stress training
- 2-week Liver and Gall Bladder Flushes
- Boxing training
- Live-In Weekend Cleanses (teach you personally how to shop consciously, clean and reorganize your kitchen and prepare Life Foods)
- Body scans and simple consultations
- Radical Life Foods Boot camp. Can you survive a weekend with the Destarchifyer?

Shout Outs and Profound Thanks to the Ever-Growing Life Foods Family

To my mentors who taught me how to heal myself
so that I might help others heal themselves.

Thank you for all of the advice and back and forth experimentation with recipes, improving our craft.

To Raw Foods Steve Melkin from Chefchaouen RIP, Ingrid from Casablanca, Luke, Thomas the Cleanser, Iris and family.

To Dr. David Jubb for his brilliance and creativity.

To the whole crew who has formed part of the journey and used a sense of humor to combat the overwhelming monotony and absurdity that surrounds us. Juan Pablo, Gammy, Louie the Plumber, Tommy, Drew, Shawn and Jenny the Empress and Emperor of the 10455 Kombucha mothership. Max, Juan Carlos, Sawyer, Jeff, Amilton e nha familia Kriola. We cannot do this alone. Let's do this as a family.

To my sons Ernesto Rafael and Caũa Amaru: I hope you have enjoyed our trips through many a kitchen as much as I have.

To all the comrades in the PSL and the wider movement: We stand before history, fully confident that we can topple this disastrous, genocidal system and build anew.

To Vinny: On July 3^{rd,} 2013 — in a blindfolded yoga session — a young man was resurrected. Your discipline and balance inspire! When my best friend and comrade embraced this disciplined way of life, I became even more potent, because now we were pushing the limits together.

To Brockton and the Bronx:
I was formed in the crucible of your flames
What didn't break me,
emboldened me.
A heir to your loyalty, grit and resistance.
Always on that hustle
I'm proud to be your son.
To fight for newly-formed horizons
where survival is guaranteed
and we can commence, at last,
to breathe
&
live free.

About the Author

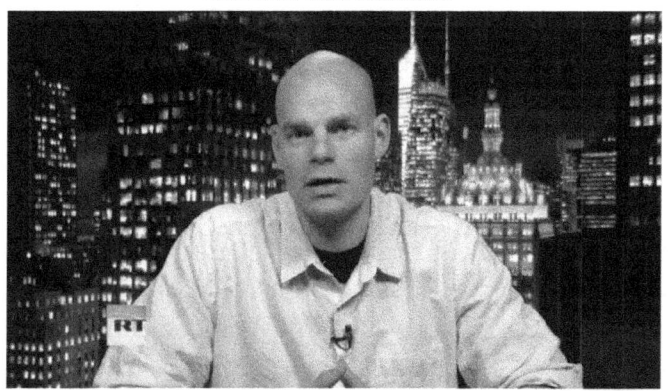

Danny Shaw teaches Latin American and Caribbean Studies and Race, Ethnicity, Class and Gender at the City University of New York. He holds a Masters in International Affairs from the School of International and Public Affairs at Columbia University. Born and raised by a single mother in Brockton, Massachusetts, he has lived in the Bronx for the past 22 years. He is fluent in Spanish, Haitian Kreyol, Portuguese, Cape Verdean Kreolu and has a fair command of French. Worked and organizing in over fifty different countries opened his spirit to countless testimonies about the inhumanity of the international economic system. A Golden Gloves boxer, he fought twice in Madison Square Garden for the NYC heavyweight championship. He teaches boxing, yoga and nutrition, working to keep young people out of the military and prison industrial complex. He is a mentor to many guiding them through the nutritional, ideological, social and emotional landmines that surround us. He is the father of two young Life Warriors, Ernesto Rafael and Cauã Amaru. A list of his other books follows: 365 Days of Resistance: We Stand on the Shoulders of Giants, Shedding that which is Not Us: A Working-Class Guide to Life Foods Training and Healing, The Saints of Santo Domingo: Dominican Resistance in the Age of Neocolonialism, My Son Blazes within Me: So Many Contradictions, So Little Time and Diving over Infinite Horizons: Journal Entries of an Internationalist. Danny has also authored blogs and articles on Latin American history, boxing and nutrition, among other topics. His contact information is DRS33@Columbia.edu.

www.ingramcontent.com/pod-product-compliance
Lightning Source LLC
Chambersburg PA
CBHW051908170526
45168CB00001B/298